# How to Cure a Cold in Two Days

## With a Breakthrough Method

**You cannot, and don't have to kill any of the 200 common cold viruses, but you can cure the common cold easily, quickly, safely, and cost-effectively once you know how.**

# by James Liu, MD, PhD
# Lilly Zhang, PhD

ISBN-13: 978-1463668365
ISBN-10: 1463668368

Publisher's Note: Neither the publisher nor the authors are engaged in providing professional medical advice or service to the individual reader. The content, ideas, procedures, and suggestions in this book are not intended as a substitute for professional medical attention. For all matters regarding your health and diseases, please consult a healthcare professional. Neither the publisher nor the authors are liable or responsible for any loss or damage allegedly arising from any material in this book. The authors and publisher are not responsible for your specific health or infection needs that may require medical supervision, nor any adverse reactions to any procedures or information provided in this book.

# Dedication

This book is dedicated to:

Our parents, who set an example of working hard and smartly in order to get the best;

Our teachers, who taught us, so we would become capable of contributing to this great society. Our PhD advisers, Dr. John A. Milner for James and Dr. John S. Bertram for Lilly, are our role models for our professional life.

Our neighbors in the global village, some close to us, some far away from us, who suffered or are suffering from the common cold, and join us in winning the war against the common cold.

**How to Use This Book**:

Depending on how urgently you need to help yourself or your loved ones to be free from the common cold, you may start to read Chapter 2 first. Chapter 2 provides information on why the common cold is a simple and curable disease.

Then, you may jump to Chapter 10. Chapter 10 details simple steps for you to cure the common cold quickly, and even how to prevent the common cold.

Chapter 11 is for those readers with certain health conditions, such as asthma, sinusitis, chronic obstructive pulmonary disease (COPD), and pregnant women with common cold, to reduce the health risk caused by cold viruses. Cleansing out viruses and bacteria out of your nasal cavities also helps to reduce bad breath.

Chapter 1 contains background information about common cold and structure of nasal cavities.

Chapter 3 shows what are those major viruses to cause the common cold.

Chapter 4 explains how the viruses and immunity to fight against each other, and therefore to cause the disease.

Chapter 5 points out why the current drug treatment of inflammation alone cannot shorten the duration of the common cold.

Chapter 6 demonstrates why the current drug treatment of inflammation alone cannot shorten the duration of the common cold.

Chapter 7 presents the clinical evidence that performing an effective nasal cleansing is profoundly effective in curing the common cold and flu.

Chapter 8 compares the advantages and disadvantages of the currently available products for performing nasal cleansing.

Chapter 9 provides the information and characteristics of the award winning product for treating cough, cold and allergy, in order for you to comprehend the advantages of using the advanced nasal irrigation system to perform an effective nasal cleansing to cure the cold.

# Contents

# Acknowledgments

This book would not have been possible without the professional guidance from our role models and the dedication of our team and family members who in one way or another contributed to the preparation and completion of this book.

Dr. John A. Milner, former President of the American Society for Nutritional Sciences, taught us how to design and conduct scientific research to improve the quality of life for men and women, young and old. That strong foundation enabled us to develop several innovative healthcare products over the past eighteen years.

Dr. Helen Guthrie, former President of the American Institute of Nutrition, encouraged and guided Dr. James Liu in designing a new method for educating the general public on how to use food to become healthy and reduce the risk of diseases. This book is the continual effort in sharing scientific knowledge with the general public.

Dr. Milo Hilty, a well-respected pediatrician in Columbus, Ohio, offered an important lesson when James Liu started working for Ross/Abbott Laboratories in 1994, when James's son was four months old: "only after you are confident that the formula is safe to feed your own baby can you start testing the new formula for other babies." This guiding principle has been extremely beneficial for us to ensure that only the safest and most effective products are offered to consumers. We believe this principle is reflected throughout this book.

The same Dr. Milo Hilty charged James Liu with a special task in 1994 to lead a strategic-clinical research team to develop the next generation of infant formula. Dr. Hilty thought that if a safe anti-infective agent was added to infant formula, babies could be protected against common upper respiratory tract infections. The alternative use of anti-infective agents by Dr. Hilty broadened our view on how to fight against pathogenic microorganisms. This book is the result of the similar alternative thinking.

Dr. Andrew T. Putney wrote a few years ago that "through my discussion with Dr. James Liu about the use of nasal irrigation for common upper respiratory infections, I have been quite excited by the possibilities for product in the primary care setting. The research I have seen on the use of "neti pots" and similar devices is quite promising. If this device can be demonstrated to limit the severity and duration of viral upper respiratory infections, it would be a godsend!" It is our wish that the device and the method presented in this book can aid family physicians like Dr. Putney in caring for their patients.

Dr. David Prezant, Chief Medical Officer for the Fire Department of the City of New York, himself inhaled toxic dust at Ground Zero when he cared for his extraordinary patients – the heroic 9/11 firefighters. Dr. Prezant objectively selected the cost-effective NasalCare® nasal irrigation products to improve the quality of life for these brave first-line responders. His medical professionalism is our own inspiration for bettering the greater society.

Our sincere gratitude is to our colleagues and friends, Dr. Wayne Zuo, Dr. Peter He, and Dr. Shane Wang, who helped us very meaningfully during the development of the NasalCare® nasal irrigation product, which is publicly recognized as the "Best New Product" at the 2010 Cough & Cold and Allergy Conference. Subsequently, medical researchers lead by Dr. Huafei Ao who used his own research funding conducted the historical clinical study, and found out that patients with either the cold or flu performed nasal irrigation three times a day can significantly reduce viral infection severity and shortened common cold duration by an average of 4.5 days. It is such a medical breakthrough that inspired us to write this book to share this safe, easy, economical and effective therapy with the public.

# 1. Understanding Common Cold and Nasal Cavities

The common cold is a viral infection of the nose. Its scientific name is viral rhinitis. Sneezing, scratchy throat, runny nose—everyone knows the first signs of a cold, probably the most common illness known. Its symptoms last 1 to 2 weeks. Children have about two to six colds a year, while adults average about one to three colds a year. Virtually everyone is familiar with the common cold.

The common cold is also the most common disease worldwide. In the US alone, the cost to the economy due to common colds was more than $40 billion dollars a year as estimated in 2003 by leading investigators at the University of Michigan Health System (Dr. Fendrick et al). This cost is substantially more than other conditions such as asthma, heart failure and emphysema. Each year, the cold leads to more than 100 million physician visits, 189 million missed school days, 126 million missed workdays for parents to stay home to care for their sick children; and millions of missed working days by employees suffering from a cold. Americans spend $2.9 billion dollars on over-the-counter drugs and another $400 million dollars on prescription medicines for symptomatic relief.

Additionally, more than $1.1 billion dollars are spent annually on the estimated 41 million dollars of antibiotic prescriptions for cold sufferers, even though antibiotics have no effect on a viral illness. It is very concerning that these treatment patterns, opposed by the CDC, contribute to the development of antibiotic resistance, a significant public health concern in addition to the economy loss. Because there was not believed to be a cure for the cold it received far less attention than many less common conditions from the pharmaceutical companies. Therefore, an intervention that would effectively prevent and/or treat the cold would have a huge health and economic impact, even greater than for chronic heart diseases.

To understand how to cure the common cold, it is helpful to know the structure and function of the nasal cavities, where cold viruses cause all kinds of problems.

In recent years, there has been an explosion of new scientific information on the structure and function of the nasal cavities at the macroscopic, microscopic, and molecular levels of analysis. The tremendous advances made over the many years in our knowledge of how humans and animals smell were highlighted by the Nobel Assembly to award the 2004 Nobel Prize in Physiology or Medicine to Dr. Richard Axel and Dr. Linda Buck for their discoveries of odorant receptors and the organization of the olfactory system. Our noses received their attention!

Currently, we have a good understanding of the cellular structure and function of the surface epithelial cells that line the nasal passages in human beings. Adverse effects may occur in the nasal epithelium after short or long exposures to various inhaled microbial, physical or chemical pathogens, like those found in living or working environments.

To maintain nasal function, the solution delivered with any nasal irrigation devices must be physiologically right--no one wants to lose their sense of smell. Every effort should be made by the manufacturer to provide, and by the customers to select, the right solution to maintain normal nasal structure and function.

## The Structure of the Nasal Cavities

The nasal cavities include the external or visible portion of the nostrils, and the cavities lying within (Figure 1-1), which are technically designated the nasal passages. It is of course the latter that are more important from a cold-therapy standpoint.

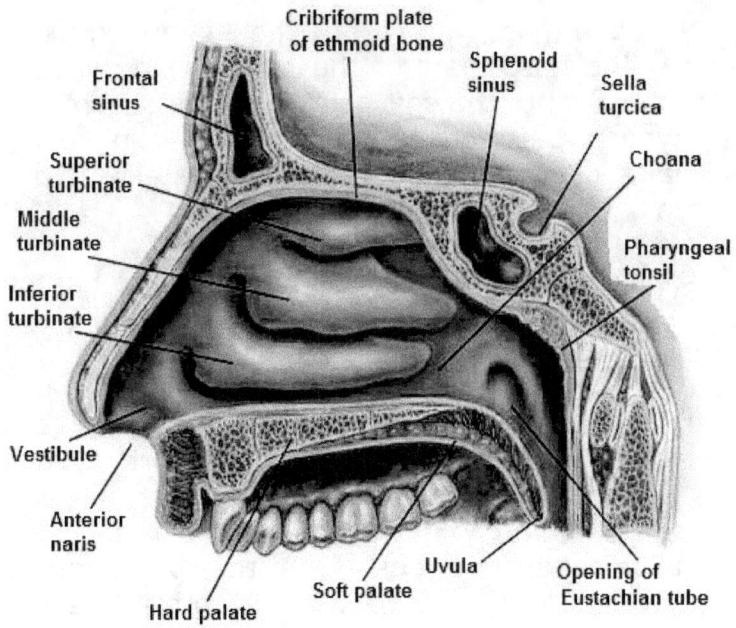

Figure 1-1. Diagram of the Nasal Cavity

## The Septum

The hollow spaces of the nasal cavity are divided into left and right sides by a vertical partition called the septum. The septum begins at the nostrils and extends backward to the posterior nares, where the left and right side to join together at the nasopharynx, the point of connection with the throat.

The septum usually deviates a little to one side or the other. When the deviation is very noticeable, it will tend to close the side of the nose to which it is inclined. When you have a cold, the blockage of air in the narrow side of the nasal cavity will be more severe.

## The Nasopharynx

As the uppermost part of the pharynx, the nasopharynx (the nasal part of the pharynx) runs from the base of the skull to the soft palate. It differs from the oral and laryngeal parts of the pharynx in that its cavity always remains open in order to communicate with the nasal cavity.

The nasopharynx is the most common place to harbor cold viruses. If further infected by bacteria, the nasopharynx is where physicians go to get a specimen for identification. Some of you may have experienced the nasal wash procedure: the doctor or nurse will inject several cc's of normal saline into the deep part of your nasal passage and then withdraw the liquid. If you have an infection, this liquid has millions of viruses or bacteria, or both. This procedure provides a clue: the specimen has so many individual viruses or bacteria or both in a small volume, such as 5 cc's. Now, think, if you ran more than 200 cc's of liquid through the nasal and nasopharyngeal cavities, more viruses or bacteria would be cleaned out!

## The Turbinates

Projecting from the outer walls of the nasal passage, there are three bony shelves—the turbinates. They have a special thick elastic network of veins, which, depending on the stimuli, will dilate and fill up with blood or completely collapse when contracted, for example, by using a drug. It is not a good idea to use  such nasal drugs too often to open up your nasal passages.

## The Eustachian Tubes

On the side walls of the nasopharynx are the openings of the Eustachian tubes, connecting with the middle ear cavities, which contain the hearing apparatus. In adults, the Eustachian tube is about 35 mm long (1.3 inches) and approximately 3 mm in diameter.

The tissue that lines the Eustachian tube is similar to that inside the nasal cavity and may have the same inflammation when presented with similar pathogenic stimuli.

For nasal irrigation, it is important to know that the pressure of the liquid flowing into the nasal cavities cannot be too high. Otherwise, the liquid may be forced into the ears through the Eustachian tubes and can cause ear pressure or ear pain. The position of your head is also important. If your head is straight, both Eustachian tubes are higher than nasopharynx, the liquid will not run into your ear. If you tilt your head to the side, as with a neti pot, the Eustachian tube of the lower ear may have a risk of letting the liquid run in.

## The Sinuses

The sinuses are four pairs of large air cavities in the bones of the face and skull. The sinuses continually secrete mucus and drain into the nose. Allergies and infections due to viruses or bacteria can cause inflammation and abscesses, or an accumulation of pus. The corresponding sinuses in each pair are symmetrical and connected with their counterparts.

### *The Frontal Sinuses*

The volume of the frontal sinus is approximately 6 to 7 milliliters (28 x 24 x 20 mm). Frontal sinus anatomy varies greatly among individuals, but generally, the two sinuses are funnel shaped and point upward. Both have their ostia (small openings) at the lowest point of the cavity. In addition, the frontal sinuses are located in the area above the eyebrows, a higher position relative to the other three pairs of sinuses, so drainage is easier. Many ear, nose, and throat doctors (ENTs) have observed that these two sinuses are rarely involved with infectious disease.

### *The Sphenoid Sinuses*

The sphenoid sinus can hold a volume of 7.5 milliliters (23 x 20 x 17 mm), and its shape varies. Generally, these sinuses are located behind the nasal cavity, though the position of the sinus and its anatomic relationships depend on the extent of hollowness. The sphenoid sinus osmium has a large opening which is narrowed by a membranous septum.

## The Ethmoid Sinuses

The ethmoid sinuses are shaped like pyramids and are divided into multiple cells by thin septa. These front and back cell spaces combined have a volume of 15 milliliters (33 x 27 x 14 mm cm). The roof of the ethmoid sinus is composed of several important structures. Because of the number and intricate disposition of the cells, these two sinuses are also called the ethmoidal labyrinth.

## The Maxillary Sinuses

Of all the sinuses, the largest are the maxillary sinuses. The adult maxillary sinus has a volume of approximately 15 milliliters (34 x 33 x 23 mm) and occupies the hollow of the cheek. Its roof corresponds to the floor of the orbit of the eye, and its floor is above the roots of the teeth, which, in fact, often penetrate into the sinus cavity. Because of the close relationship between the sinuses and the type, number, and arrangement of the teeth, dental disease can cause maxillary sinus infection, and tooth extraction can result in oral-antral fistulae, abnormal passageways from the mouth to the maxillary sinus. By the age of nine, in humans, the floor of the maxillary sinus is generally at the level of the nasal floor. The floor continues to sink as the maxillary sinus becomes more air-filled as a person matures. Therefore, it is understandable that when people perform nasal irrigation, there will be certain amount of liquid remaining in these two sinuses because their position is lower than the nasal floor. Because they occupy the lowest position of all sinuses, the maxillary sinuses have the highest chance of becoming infected, and these infections are also hard to treat. When you perform a nasal irrigation, some liquid may remain this sinus.

## The Mucous Membrane of Nasal Cavity

The mucous membrane lining the interior of the nasal cavity extends through the little pathways of communication to line the accessory sinuses, so that it is easy for disease to spread from the nasal passages into the nasal sinuses and vice versa. It is supplied with numerous minute glands that open on its free surface, some of which create the ever-present secretions. The glands are of two kinds: mucous, which secrete a thick and sticky substance, and serous glands, which secrete a thin watery fluid.

The nasal mucous membrane is richly supplied with blood vessels and nerves. The nerves are of three kinds:

1) sensory, those that have to do with common sensation;
2) sympathetic, those that have control of the veins of the swelling tissue, and
3) olfactory, the nerve that serves the function of the special sense of smell.

The first kind is evident in the extreme sensitivity of the nose; its marked irritability, as shown by a tendency "to run" and to cause sneezing with slight provocation, is due to the unique distribution of nerves of common sensation.

The second kind is present in a small ganglion of the sympathetic system, called Meckel's ganglion, which is situated in the upper part of the nose. These give rise to the vasomotor nerves, which control the network of veins constituting the erectile tissue. Responding to certain stimuli, therefore, the vasomotor nerves of the nose acting upon these vessels will cause them to contract and dilate according to physiological needs.

Third, we have the olfactory nerve or special nerve for the sense of smell. Just before entering the nose, it breaks up into a number of threads, which perforate the roof of the nose through little openings in the cribriform plate and pass downward to supply the mucus membrane. The olfactory nerve is not supplied to the entire mucus membrane of the nose, as some suppose, but to a very limited area in the uppermost part. This smelling area has been found to extend only as far as the upper margin of the middle turbinal, and a corresponding surface on the septum.

## The Oral Cavity

The oral cavity is so closely connected to the nasal cavity that when one experiences a viral attack, the other feels the pain. With the common cold, the primary infection occurs in the nasal cavity, but the oral cavity demonstrates the early symptoms, such as a sore throat. Simply put, the inflammatory secretion comes out of the nasal cavity and flows directly down into the throat. The throat is then irritated and inflamed, and sends the signal to the body to pay attention.

## The Oropharynx

As distinguished from the nasopharynx, the part of the throat we see when we look directly in through the open mouth is called the pharynx, or more properly, the oropharynx, an important part of the oral cavity.

Still lower, we have the part just back of the larynx, called the laryngopharynx, which continues on down into the esophagus, while the continuation of the air tract is represented by the larynx and the trachea, which lies just in front.

## The Soft Palate

As we look into the throat, we see a sort of curtain suspended from the roof of the mouth, the lower borders of which form two half arches meeting in the middle. This is the soft palate, and its central downward prolongation constitutes the uvula. Together, they mark the boundary between the pharynx and the mouth. The soft palate is made up largely of muscle, as evidenced by the contracting action you see when a person utters the sound "ah"; the palate becomes elevated, and the uvula contracts almost out of sight.

The name *hard palate* is applied to the entire arched roof of the mouth, which is a bony formation. It is limited by the gums (alveolar process) in front and on the side and ends posteriorly in a free border to which the soft palate is attached.

## The Tonsils

The two palatine (faucial) tonsils are almond-shaped bodies measuring about 1.0 by 0.5 inches (25 by 12 millimeters) and are embedded between the folds of tissue connecting the pharynx and the posterior part of the tongue with the soft palate. The lingual tonsil occupies the posterior part of the tongue surface. It is really a collection of 35 to 100 separate tonsillar units, each having a single crypt surrounded by lymphoid tissue. Each tonsil forms a smooth swelling about 0.08 to 0.16 inches (2 to 4 millimeters) in diameter. The pharyngeal tonsil (called adenoids when enlarged) occupies the roof of the nasal part of the pharynx. This tonsil may enlarge during a cold viral infection to block the nasal passage, forcing the person to breathe through the mouth.

The tonsils are the important local sources of blood lymphocytes. They often become inflamed and enlarged during a cold. If the tonsil inflammation becomes chronic, it may be necessary to have them surgically removed.

## The Function of the Nasal Cavity

The nasal cavity conditions the air to be received by the other areas of the respiratory tract, mainly, the lung. Owing to the large surface area provided by the turbinates, the air passing through the nasal cavity is warmed or cooled to within one degree of the body temperature. In addition, the air is humidified, and dust and other particulate matter is removed by cilia vibrates, which are short, thick hairs in the vestibule. The cilia of the respiratory epithelium move the particulate matter toward the pharynx, where it passes into the esophagus and is digested in the stomach.

Cilia and mucus along the inside wall of the nasal cavity trap and remove dust and pathogens from the air as it flows through the nasal cavity. The cilia move the mucus down the nasal cavity to the pharynx, where it can be swallowed.

The nasal cavity is divided into two segments: the respiratory segment and the olfactory segment.

## Breathing

The respiratory segment of the nasal cavity is lined with respiratory epithelium. It also has a very rich vascular structure, allowing the venous network of the conchal (turbinate) mucosa to engorge with blood, which restricts airflow and causes the air to be directed to the other side of the nose. This cycle occurs approximately every twenty to thirty minutes.

The most important and primary function of the respiratory system is to supply oxygen to the body's cells. During inhalation, air is drawn from the atmosphere, through the nose (sometimes, through mouth too). This is caused by the contraction of the diaphragm (the sheet of muscles that separate the thoracic cavity from the abdominal cavity) and the intercostal muscles attached to the ribs. As they contract, the volume of the thoracic cavity increases, thereby decreasing the air pressure, resulting in inhalation.

The air taken through the nose is filtered, moistened, and heated in the nasal cavity, before it passes to the pharynx. The pharynx's function is to facilitate the passage of air to the trachea. The flap-like structure (called the epiglottis), located just above the opening, closes this orifice when food is swallowed, ensuring that food particles do not enter the trachea. It is near this opening that the voice box or the larynx is situated. This structure performs the function of protecting the trachea and producing the sounds for speech.

**The Sense of Smell**

The olfactory segment of the nasal cavity is lined with a specialized type of olfactory epithelium, which contains receptors for scents. In humans, the olfactory epithelium measures about 1 square centimeter (on each side) and lies on the roof of the nasal cavity about 7 centimeters above and behind the nostrils. The olfactory epithelium is the part of the olfactory system directly responsible for detecting odors.

## Olfactory Cells

The olfactory cells of the epithelium are bipolar neurons that congregate to form the olfactory nerve. The apical poles (at each end) of these neurons are covered with nonmotile cilia. The plasma membrane contains the odorant-binding proteins that act as olfactory receptors. The incoming odorants are made soluble by the serous secretion from the Bowman's glands, which are located in the lamina propria of the mucosa.

## Supporting Cells

The supporting cells of the olfactory epithelium function as metabolic and physical support for the olfactory cells. Histologically (in terms of tissue structure), the supporting cells are tall, columnar cells featuring microvilli and a prominent terminal web. The nuclei of supporting cells are more apically located than those of the other olfactory epithelial cells.

## Basal Cells

Basal cells rest on the basal lamina of the olfactory epithelium; these cells are stem cells capable of division and differentiation into either supporting or olfactory cells. The constant divisions of the basal cells lead to the olfactory epithelium being replaced every two to four weeks. Basal cells can be divided on the basis of cellular anatomy histological markers into two populations: the horizontal basal cells, which line the olfactory epithelium, and the slightly more superficial globose basal cells. Horizontal basal cells are now thought to be the primary stem cell population supplying new cells to this system, although this is still subject to some debate, with some scientists maintaining that the globose basal cells are the true stem cells.

## Brush Cells

Brush cells are microvilli-bearing columnar cells with a basal surface in contact with the afferent nerve endings. They are specialized for the transduction of general sensation. The nerve fibers are terminal branches of the trigeminal nerve (cranial nerve V), rather than the olfactory nerve, as afferent olfactory signals are.

## Olfactory Glands

Tubuloalveolar serous secreting glands lie in the lamina propria of the mucosa. These glands deliver a proteinaceous secretion via ducts onto the surface of the mucosa. The role of the secretions is to trap and dissolve odiferous substances for the bipolar neurons. The constant flow from the olfactory glands allows old odors to be constantly washed away.

## Pathology

The olfactory epithelium can be damaged by inhalation of toxic fumes, physical injury to the interior of the nose, and possibly by the use of some nasal sprays or the wrong nasal irrigation liquid. Because of its regenerative capacity, damage to the olfactory epithelium is usually temporary, but in extreme cases, injury can be permanent, leading to anosmia.

## 2. The Common Cold Is a Simple Disease

Every disease is different. Some diseases are very complicated, such as diabetes. With diabetes, virtually the whole body—all the organs and all the tissues—are involved. Many diabetic patients have abnormalities in multiple organs and body parts, including the eyes, heart, kidneys, legs, and others. To treat diabetes, the patient must rely on a specially trained medical expert—an endocrinologist. This special doctor prescribes the right drugs to meet the individual patient's needs. Since all of these organs and tissues will be influenced, the choice of drug has a long-term influence on the body.

However, some diseases are relatively simple, such as a spinal disc herniation. Anyone who has had a herniated spinal disc in the neck or the back knows what it means in terms of neck or back pain. Although the consequences are very severe, the disease itself is a local problem. It is a not a condition the patient can fix on his or her own. A very skilled doctor is required to fix the herniated disc.

Other diseases are even simpler, such as the common cold; only cold viruses cause this kind of damage, and the problem is mainly in the nose. For the common cold, however, your doctors currently have no antiviral drugs to help you, so you have to cure yourself. Since the common cold is a simple disease, you can focus on your nasal cavities, not the other parts of the body. After you read this book, you will be able to cure your own cold safely, easily, effectively, quickly, and economically.

You may be disagreeing with us right now. You've no doubt heard that the common cold is not that simple. Any of more than two hundred different viruses can cause a cold, and even after you get a cold, your immunity against another cold is very limited, since any of the other two hundred plus viruses can give you a new cold. And you are right. In some ways, the common cold is a very challenging disease. In addition, there is no vaccine available to prevent infection from any of these common cold viruses. In spite of these facts, we still say the common cold a very simple disease–let us explain why.

## The Root Cause of the Common Cold Is Clear

The virus causes the common cold and is one of over two hundred cold viruses. Without a virus to trigger the infection in the nasal cavity, the common cold cannot arise. It must replicate to have a large enough population to cause the symptomatic disease. To win the battle against the cold virus, you must stop the virus's growth.

A viral infection is very different from a toxin-caused disorder. Unlike a toxin-induced reaction, the cold virus–caused disease is not that acute. For the common cold, it takes one to three days after catching a cold virus to have symptoms--the incubation period. They start with a burning feeling in the nose or throat. Next comes sneezing, a runny nose, and the feeling of being tired and unwell.

There are several factors that make you more susceptible to a cold virus. For example, you are more likely to catch a common cold when you, the host, are excessively fatigued, have emotional distress, or have allergies with nose and throat symptoms. But, no matter what else, introducing cold viruses into your nasal cavities from the environment contaminated by the patients carrying viruses is the key step. These three-way interrelationships are presented in Figure 2-1. When you are "down" and easy to be infected, if you inhaled in the air or touched a door knob contaminated with cold viruses , you can develop a common cold.

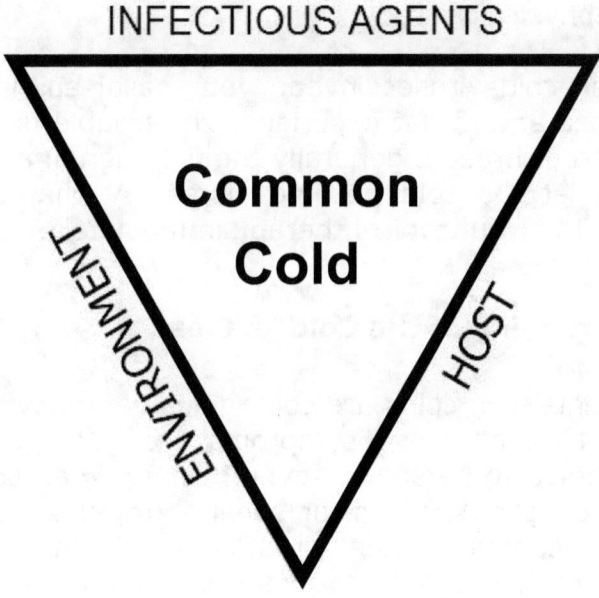

Figure 2-1. Relationship among viruses, spreading in the environment and human body as the host.

## The Location of the Cold Disease Is Clear

The cold virus grows at 91° F (33° C), making your nose and throat the perfect place for these viruses to grow (Couch RB. Rhinoviruses. In: Fields Virology 1996). That's why the common cold is also called viral rhinitis (the root *rhin-* meaning "nose"). The common cold is truly a nasal disease. These viruses are not transferred through the blood. These viruses do not penetrate deeply into other tissues or organs. In addition, the damage to your nasal cavity is clearly on the surface. All of these factors provide a great possibility to have a very effective topical-physical therapy.

When cold viruses invade your nasal epithelial cells, your nose and throat experience the trouble first. That is why a sore throat is generally the first sign of a cold. Why wait to let the cold become worse? At that time, you should start your topical therapy immediately.

## The Spreading of the Cold Is Clear

Patients with colds are contagious before symptomatic infection till all these symptoms are gone. Colds pass from person to person in several ways. When an infected person coughs, sneezes, or speaks, tiny fluid droplets or aerosols containing the virus are expelled Figure 2-2. These droplets or aerosols can be breathed in by other people, then cause the new infection in their noses and airways.

Colds may also be passed through direct contact. If a person with a cold touches his runny nose or watery eyes, then shakes hands with another person, some of the viruses is transferred to the uninfected person. If that person then touches his mouth, nose, or eyes, the virus is transferred to an environment where it can reproduce and cause a cold.

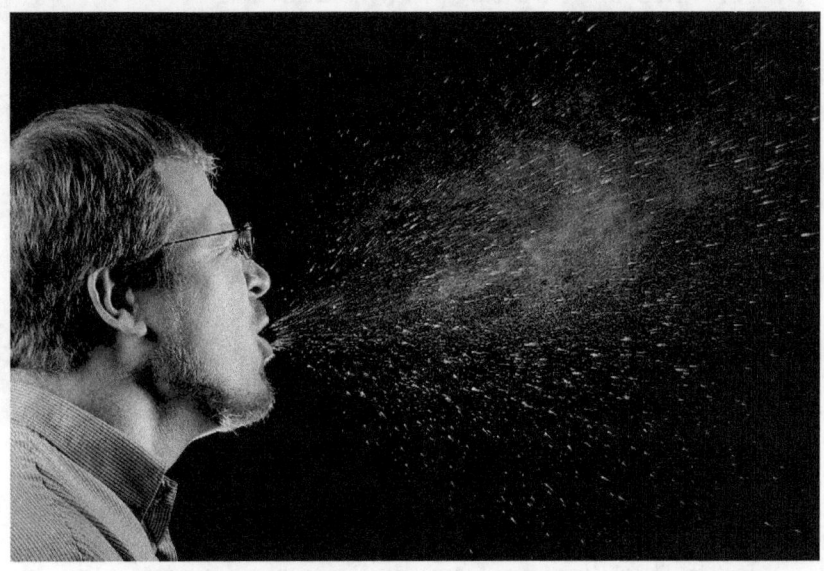

Figure 2-2. Cough-sneeze spreads viruses far and large*

*Authored by James Gathany and originally published by Center for Disease Control and Prevention.

## The Cold Disease Process Is Clear

When cold viruses invade the epithelial cells in your nasal cavity, they grow to make more. Your body's immune system sends in as many disease fighters as possible and launches all kinds of weapons to stop the viral growth. The fighting results in an inflammation. Inflammation, including edema (swelling), redness, and the extra secretions coming out of your nose are the reasons you get a sore throat, nasal congestion, sneeze, cough, and other symptoms. Therefore, the symptoms are the results of a simple battle between the virus and your body's immune system through inflammation. Figure 2-3 shows you how the cold viruses and your immune system interact through inflammation.

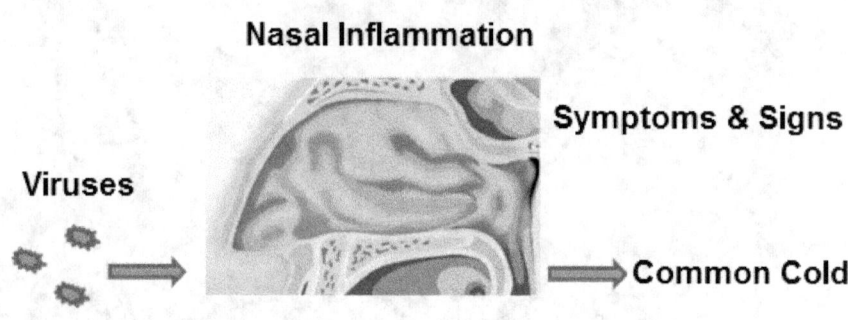

Figure 2-3. The Key Elements of a Common Cold

From this diagram, you can see that when cold viruses in the air are inhaled into your nasal cavity or introduced by a hand contaminated with cold viruses touching your nose or eye, the viruses can grow in your nasal cavity. Soon, your body's immune system detects that something's wrong, and it starts to fight back. The goal of the fight is to get rid of the cold viruses. However, the fight also causes redness, swelling, and pain in your nasal cavity. This process is commonly known as inflammation. Yes, inflammation is caused by both the cold virus and your immune response.

## The Diagnosis of a Cold Is Not Hard

During the initial stage of invasion and growth of cold viruses, your body's immune system has a minor reaction. It is so mild that you may not feel anything is wrong. When the magnitude of inflammation, the fire in your nose and throat, becomes bigger, the inflammatory secretion, or mucus, runs down to your throat. You have a sore throat at an early stage, and then you will start coughing and sneezing and feeling the nasal congestion. That is when you know you have a cold. Most people have had the cold experience many times. Here is a list of the common symptoms of a cold:

- Sore throat—The viral infection and inflammation occurs in the throat during the cold. Sore throats can be painful and annoying. You can see yourself if your throat is abnormally red.

- Cough—The thick mucus produced during a cold virus infection will drip down into the throat and upper chest, thus causing a cough.

- Sneezing—A sneeze is a strong, sudden, uncontrolled burst of air through the nose and mouth. Sneezing is caused by an irritation to the nasal lining or the throat from the mucus generated by a cold viral infection.

- Nasal congestion—The blockage of the nasal passages is due to membranes lining the nose becoming swollen from inflamed blood vessels. Nasal congestion can interfere with hearing and speech. Significant congestion may interfere with sleep, cause snoring, and be associated with sleep apnea.

It is not hard for you to self-diagnose a cold. Yes, the diagnosis of a disease should usually be made by a physician, but for the common cold, most often you are pretty accurate. You've experienced this common disease many times in the past. Every family has an accumulated knowledge of the common cold, gained over generations, and there really has not been much change in treating the common cold for hundreds of years.

It is also helpful if you know you recently came into contact with someone who had a cough or was sneezing not too far away from you. Knowledge of this close contact is particularly important for a self-diagnosis if this happens in the cold season. If you have any doubt, you should consult with your physician.

## The Treatment of a Cold Has a Clear Target

The surface of the nasal cavity is the main place for the cold viruses to grow. And the surface of the nasal cavity is the place for your immune response to fight against the viral growth. Therefore, the surface of the nasal cavity is the place you will have inflammation. The treatment target then is to eliminate viruses on the surface of the nasal cavity and, as a result, to reduce the need for the inflammatory reaction in the same place.

Now you have a good idea of where you should pay attention to when you consider ways to cure your cold, or when you contact someone with common cold symptoms in the near future, you know the target for prevention and treatment, is your nose.

Simply, no viruses in your nose means no common cold. Though knowledge is power, sadly, the increased knowledge about the cold had not added much to curing the virus infection in the past. Even as knowledgeable as medical doctors were, they had no antiviral drug to cure the common cold.

Now, however, you are living in a medicine-advanced world. The new knowledge shared in the following chapters will help you to cure the common cold by yourself safely, quickly, and economically. In the next few chapters, you will learn the details of these cold viruses, why you have the cold symptoms, what the new medical breakthrough research shows, how to select the right product for treating your common cold, and how to use the product. You will become an expert on curing the common cold quickly and easily.

Yes, the common cold is curable! And, this can be done by yourself easily.

United, we can win the war against our common enemy – the common cold.

# 3. Viruses Are the Root Cause of the Common Cold

In order to cure your cold, it is a good idea to know the root cause of the common cold disease. For any individual patient with a cold, one specific virus is generally the original troublemaker. In humans, more than two hundred different viruses cause the common cold. Among them, rhinoviruses (nasal viruses) account for about 30 to 50 percent; coronaviruses account for about 15 to 30 percent; influenza viruses account for about 5 to 15 percent. These three major groups of viruses together account for about 75 to 95 percent of all common colds. The rest of the common colds are caused by human parainfluenza viruses, human respiratory syncytial viruses, adenoviruses, enteroviruses, and metapneumoviruses. Each of these groups of viruses has subtypes. Because so many different viruses are the root cause of the common cold in the human population, it would be very difficult to develop a vaccine to prevent the common cold. Although many pharmaceutical companies have tried to develop antiviral drugs, none has been approved to treat the common cold. A new discovery made at the Massachusetts Institute of Technology (MIT) in July 2011 provides some hope of treating all cold viruses. Since the MIT advancement is made so recently, it may take many more years to develop it into a drug, and only if all clinical studies support its safety and antiviral activity.

As an individual patient with a common cold, you are most likely dealing with one type of common cold virus, not all two hundred different types of cold viruses. But pharmaceutical companies, as you can understand, have to consider that patients as a group are infected with many types of cold viruses. For economic reasons, any vaccine or antiviral drug must be useful for a relatively large patient population. Following is a brief overview of the major cold viruses.

## Rhinovirus

First, let's look at the rhinovirus (Figure 3-1), since there is about a 50 percent chance of your infection being caused by any of this group of viruses. Rhinovirus grows at 91°F (33°C). The normal temperature of the rest of your body is about 98ºF (37ºC), so the cold virus would have a hard time trying to grow in a non-nasal environment.

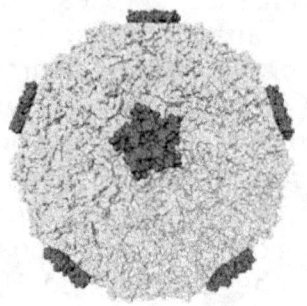

Figure 3-1. Diagram of Rhinovirus

This largely explains why the common cold is a disease of the nasal cavity. Your nose, all year round, is the preferred place for rhinovirus to grow, since the local temperature is right for it. You know, however, that more people catch colds in the winter, and that is why it's named.

Why more colds in winter than in summer? When absolute humidity is low, influenza virus survival is prolonged and transmission rates go up (Shaman, http://blogs.discovermagazine.com/80beats/2009/02/10/scientists-solve-the-mystery-of-flu-season/.
Since the virus can survive longer in cold, dry conditions, the chances are greater that someone will come along and be infected with the virus.

During winter, people are more closely in contact with other people than in the summer. You get rhinovirus from others when you inhale what was coughed or sneezed out or touch some cold-virus contaminated area with your hands.

Your contaminated hand is very likely to touch your nose. That's why your nasal cavity is where the cold virus enters your body and why it is also the location for the inflammation reaction—the cold disease.

In the nasal cavity, these rhinoviruses only grow on the surface of the nasal lining; they do not penetrate deeply into the muscle or bone. Your nasal tissue damage also happens only on the surface (epithelium). Knowing the location for most common viruses to cause a cold, you now have a clear target to pay attention to: your nasal cavity's inner surface.

## Coronaviruses

Coronaviruses are the second most frequent cause of the common cold, as they account for 15 to 30 percent of proven viral infections. Medical researchers have difficulty growing coronaviruses in the laboratory. Artificial infections of coronaviruses in volunteers has provided very useful information though. It takes three days to feel cold symptoms after the coronavirus is introduced into the nasal cavity. Significant damage to the nasal epithelium occurs following nasal infection with coronavirus. Disorders of the nasal epithelium and the functioning of nasal ciliary were found in the volunteers. Again, you have a clear target to aim toward in curing your common cold by paying attention to your nasal cavity's inner surface.

## Influenza Viruses

The number-three most common cause of the common cold is the influenza virus. You know influenza viruses are the root cause of influenza, or the flu. Colds and the flu are common infections, especially during the winter months. These infections share many of the same features. Both cold and flu are caused by viruses, and both are highly contagious. Medical research shows that when cold and influenza viruses are introduced into the nasal cavity by aerosol or by contact with saliva or other respiratory secretions from an infected individual, they attach to and replicate in the epithelial cells. Viral replication combined with the inflammation lead to the destruction and loss of cells lining the respiratory tract. Because of these similarities, the terms "flu" and "cold" are often used together. However, there are important differences between these two types of infection. Cold viruses almost never grow outside the upper respiratory tract (nasal cavity) because of their temperature sensitivity, but influenza viruses can grow both in the upper respiratory tract (nasal cavities) and lower respiratory tract (lungs). Symptoms of flu are much severer than those of a cold. Muscle pain and fever rarely accompany a cold, but often do the flu.

Medical doctors can give you a drug to treat the flu, and a flu vaccine is an option for prevention. However, if you start to have symptoms of an upper respiratory tract infection, you are more likely to have a cold, not the flu, because there is a much higher chance of catching a cold than the flu.

Whenever you have a severe infection, you should seek help from a physician. When the symptoms are minimal at the beginning of the viral infection, you cannot tell the difference between a cold and the flu. At the early stages of the viral infection, even your doctor cannot make a clear diagnosis before a viral test is done. A newly published clinical study in June 2011 clearly showed that performing nasal irrigation with the NasalCare® Nasal Irrigation Kit can effectively remove influenza viruses, and the patient quickly recovered.

Hence, it is important to start effective nasal irrigation with a pump irrigator right away, no matter whether it is cold or influenza viruses that are starting to infect your nasal cavities.

## Parainfluenza Viruses

Parainfluenza viruses (HPIV) are common causes of respiratory tract disease in infants and young children. Each of the four types of HPIVs has different clinical and epidemiologic features. The most distinctive clinical feature of HPIV-1 and HPIV-2 is croup (swelling around the vocal chords and other parts of the upper and middle airway); HPIV-3 is more often associated with bronchiolitis (swelling of the small airways leading to the lungs) and pneumonia. HPIV-4 is detected infrequently and is less likely to cause severe disease (however, it may be more common than once thought).

HPIVs can cause repeated infections throughout life, usually manifested by a cold. HPIVs can also cause serious lower respiratory tract disease with repeat infection (e.g., pneumonia, bronchitis, and bronchiolitis), especially among older adults and patients with compromised immune systems. The incubation period (time from exposure to the virus to the onset of symptoms) for HPIVs generally ranges from two to seven days. This provides a window of opportunity to clean them out before they can cause a symptomatic infection.

**Respiratory Syncytial Virus**

In adults, Respiratory syncytial virus (RSV), may only produce symptoms of the common cold, such as a stuffy or runny nose, sore throat, mild headache, cough, fever, and a general feeling of being ill. However, this virus is a major cause of respiratory illness in young children. In premature babies and kids with diseases that affect the lungs, heart, or immune system, RSV infections can lead to other more serious illnesses.

RSV is highly contagious and can be spread through droplets containing the virus expelled into the air when someone coughs or sneezes. It also can live on surfaces (such as countertops or doorknobs) and on hands and clothing and so can be easily spread when a person touches something contaminated. RSV can spread rapidly through schools and child-care centers. Babies often get it when older kids carry the virus home from school and pass it to them. Almost all kids are infected with RSV at least once by the time they're two years old. RSV infections often occur in epidemics that last from late fall through early spring. Respiratory illnesses caused by RSV—such as bronchiolitis or pneumonia—usually last about a week, but some cases may last several weeks.

Because RSV can be easily spread by touching infected people or surfaces, frequent hand-washing is key in preventing its transmission. Try to wash your hands after having any contact with someone who has cold symptoms. And keep your school-age child with a cold away from younger siblings—particularly infants—until the symptoms pass.

**Adenoviruses**

Adenovirus infections most commonly cause diseases of the respiratory system; however, depending on the infecting viral serotype, they may also cause various other illnesses, such as gastroenteritis, conjunctivitis, cystitis, and rashes. Symptoms of adenovirus infection range from the common cold syndrome to pneumonia, croup, and bronchitis. Patients with compromised immune systems are especially prone to severe complications of adenovirus infection. Acute respiratory disease (ARD), first recognized among military recruits during World War II, can be caused by adenovirus infections during conditions of crowding and stress.

After you know that these important viruses are the common root causes of the common cold, you may not need to spend a lot of time learning about the other cold viruses. As the basic infection and inflammation occur in the nasal cavity, you know your nasal cavity should be the central focus of attention, as it is the place for the viral infection and the inflammatory reaction from the body's immune system.

## Why There Is No Vaccine for Preventing Cold Virus Infection

Vaccines are very effective for preventing certain viral infections. Currently, unfortunately, there is no vaccine for the common cold. This is largely because more than 200 cold viruses can cause the cold, and it is hard to make a vaccine to target so many viruses. Scientists are searching for better methods to produce the vaccine, and it will take many years to reach success.

## Why There Are No Drugs to Treat Cold Virus Infection

Like antibiotics for treating specific bacteria, specific antiviral drugs are used for specific viruses. Currently, regrettably, there are no anti-viral drugs to treat the common cold. As with the difficulty in creating a vaccine, it is hard to develop the drug to cure the cold that is caused by many kinds of cold viruses.

# 4. Viruses and Immunity Form a Battlefield in the Nose

To cure your cold fast, you need to know how to fight against your enemy. You probably already have a general idea about what happens on a battlefield. In a battlefield, one of the commonly used approaches to win is to increase the number of fighters.

## Overgrowth of Cold Viruses

When the cold viruses invade your nasal cavity, your immune system starts to defend your body. In this unique battlefield, the virus tries to supply as many fighters as possible by growing more and more viruses in the epithelial cells of your nasal cavity. After the new generation of cold viruses is produced, they are released by breaking out of their womb—your epithelial cells! Then, these new viruses invade the nearby epithelial cells in your nasal cavity. This cycle happens again and again.

Since it is clear that the result of cold virus growth is the destruction of the epithelial cells in your nasal cavity, let's look at what is happening on the other side of the battlefield—your body's immune system. The body's immune response is comprised of many fighters, like white blood cells. When the battlefield is formed in your nose, your body can supply unlimited fighters – white blood cells.

Depending on your age, health conditions, nutritional status, and other factors, the strength of your immune response may be relatively different from others'. However, you don't need to worry about how strong your immune system is, since virtually everyone catches a cold once in any given year. Rather, it is necessary to see how your immune system fights against cold viruses.

## Immunity

Everyone has two types of immunity: the specific immunity and the nonspecific immunity.

### *Specific Immunity*

Let's review specific immunity first. It comes mainly from antibodies and lymph cells (lymphocytes) specifically target against the cold virus. These antibodies and lymphocytes only attack the cold viruses that have previously infected you. They do not have any memory of the other types of cold viruses since they have not previously infected you. In helping you to win the battle against the current cold viruses, the specific immunity is generally very weakly, if at all, effective during the early phase of the fighting. Why? Basically, not many of these specific antibodies and lymphocytes are there when your body is invaded by the cold viruses. The specific immunity has about two years of memory for a specific virus—one of the two hundred viruses. After two years, the memory for that specific virus is gone. The functional-specific antibodies and lymphocytes are reproduced for about two weeks after you contract the current infection. By that time, your cold symptoms generally disappear if you are not further infected by bacteria. Therefore, you cannot count on your specific immunity to help you fight against current cold viruses. The good thing is that the newly-gained specific immunity helps you to prevent the same cold virus from invading your body again in the next two years. Your specific immunity does not cause you any harm during the two weeks of cold, as it is not a noticeable player on the battlefield. Because of their number, they basically don't participate in the inflammation reactions for the first two weeks.

It may be beneficial to briefly share the process of antibody production in our body. When particles of a cold virus enter our nose and are identified by the immune system as foreign "invaders", our bodies use the invaders, which are also called antigens, as a template to create a genetically matching antibodies. Antibodies, also known as immunoglobulins, are like a lock and key system with the specific virus. When matched perfectly with the cold virus antigens, they "lock" or bind the antigens, neutralizing them so they can no longer enter or damage our epithelial cells in nasal cavities. To bind each different strain of cold viruses, the antibodies must have the right pattern to match the characteristics of each antigen. A match will allow the antibodies and immune response to make a "lock" to fit those viruses. Our body remembers each new virus pattern that has caused an immune response in the past, so that it can make those matching cells to protect us from that same specific cold/flu strain in case it ever enters the body again in the future.

Our body has the ability to determine when a cold or flu virus has invaded and, if it has a match to that strain of virus stored from a prior invasion, the immune response is generated and the immune system (white blood cells) quickly  produce a lot of those antibodies, that the body made and that worked in the past to destroy/bind the invading virus particles. If it is a new invading virus, usually our body can make cells that can match just right in a week to ten days. However, if the new invading virus is a new one, our body cannot make any antibodies to against it.

## *Nonspecific Immunity*

The other type of immunity is called nonspecific immunity. Nonspecific immunity has many powerful fighters to help you win the battle against cold viruses.

The frontline fighters of nonspecific immunity are the big white blood cells called macrophages. They are near the epithelial cells that have been infected by cold viruses. A macrophage is a specific type of white blood cell that ingests (takes in) foreign material. Macrophages are key players in the immune response to foreign invaders like cold viruses. The macrophage has its own supplier in the blood monocytes, a particular type of white blood cells. Monocytes migrate into the virus-invaded epithelium in the nasal cavity, and there they differentiate (evolve) into macrophages. Macrophages help destroy viruses, bacteria, and protozoa when a complicated infection occurs. Macrophages serve as scavengers that rid the body of worn-out cells and other debris. Their other, more important role is to release biological signals to initiate the inflammation reaction.

If you have ever burned or cut yourself, you might have observed inflammation in the damaged tissue. You saw swelling and redness and felt heat and pain. Swelling is caused by the creation of gaps between the capillary cells, allowing the movement of fluid and immune cells to the damaged area. An increase in blood flow to the area causes the characteristic redness. Heat is caused by the accumulation of blood and the release of fever-inducing molecules called pyrogens. Pain is felt in response to tissue damage and the irritation of sensory nerves in the affected area. This series of events is collectively called "inflammation." That is happening in your nasal cavity when you have a common cold. When you open your mouth to say "Ahh" in front of a mirror, you can see the redness of your throat. When the swelling occurs in your internal nasal cavity, you can feel the nasal congestion.

## Inflammation

The English word *inflammation* comes from the Latin *inflammare*, which means "to set on fire." Inflammation is a biological fire in the human body. It is part of the complex biological response of vascular tissues to harmful stimuli, such as viruses and damaged cells at the cold-virus infected site. Inflammation occurs to remove the injurious stimuli and to initiate the healing process. However, progressive destruction caused by inflammation of the tissue is part of the virus-triggered nasal lining damage. In addition, unwanted inflammation can also be a major destructive force, as seen in many autoimmune diseases. It is for that reason that inflammation is normally closely regulated by the body.

There are significant side effects from inflammation, but your body needs it to fight against cold viruses. Inflammation is like a toxic but essential drug: Although the drug causes significant side effects, you will take it if you need the drug to save your life. This is more or less like what happens on a battlefield: no matter which side fires the bullets or drops the bombs, the surrounding area gets damaged. Many powerful and destructive inflammatory mediators are released by your immune system. They attack viruses and damage your own cells.

To fight against common cold viruses, so far modern medicine's approach is still similar to what was done in the pre-penicillin age against bacterial infections. Unless and until an antiviral drug is available, you must suffer the inflammation to save your life. However, in a later chapter, you will learn about a new method to fight against cold virus infections, which will make you less dependent on inflammation to cure colds.

Your goal is to stop the activities on the battlefield of your nasal cavities from ever occurring. These damaging attacks and counterattacks are happening in your nasal cavity and cause you to suffer greatly.

## Coughing and Sneezing the Cold Virus Out

Coughing and sneezing are the body's way of removing viruses or mucus from the nasal cavity and lungs. A cough is only a symptom, not a disease. A productive cough produces mucus and generally it should not be suppressed. It clears virus-laden mucus from the nasal cavity and lungs. On the negative side, coughing and sneezing are a major way of spreading viruses around.

A nonproductive cough is dry and does not produce sputum. A dry, hacking cough may develop toward the end of a cold. A chronic dry cough may be a sign of mild asthma, since many times, an asthma attack follows an infection by cold viruses. Nonproductive coughing does not help to get rid of viruses.

Coughing can only play a very limited role in removing cold viruses. Therefore, no matter how productive it is, you must use a more effective method to get rid of the cold viruses in your body.

# 5. Suppressing Inflammation Alone Cannot Cure a Cold

From the previous chapter, you know that the symptoms of a cold are not caused by the virus alone, as virus growth itself is very small. The symptoms of a cold are due to the body's inflammatory response. Chemical agents manufactured by our immune system inflame our cells and tissues, causing our nose to run and our throat to swell. The damage largely is from our own immune system fighting with the viruses.

It is possible to create the full storm of cold symptoms with no cold virus at all. A potent cocktail of the inflammatory mediators is made by the body's immune system. It includes cytokines, kinins, prostaglandins, and interleukins, all powerful little chemical messengers. These inflammatory mediators cause blood vessels in the nose to dilate and leak, stimulate the secretion of mucus, activate sneeze and cough reflexes, and set off pain in our nerve fibers.

Contrary to general wisdom, our tendency to have bad cold symptoms is not a sign of a weakened immune system—quite the opposite in fact. Pharmaceutical research has figured out that anti-inflammation drugs are effective in treating colds. If you try to strengthen your immune system, it may be counterproductive. It could aggravate the symptoms by amplifying the very inflammatory agents that caused them in the first place. That means that a stronger immune system can call for more micro-fighters to release more bullets and bombs in the battlefields of your nasal cavity.

Several anti-inflammatory approaches have been used to alleviate cold symptoms. Let's review them.

## Chicken Soup

Homemade chicken soup has long been used to fight the common cold. It flushes out the nasal passages with its aromatic steam and offers hydration and comfort.

There is evidence that chicken soup has anti-inflammatory properties, particularly if the skin is left in. In 2000, scientists at the University of Nebraska Medical Center in Omaha found that some components of chicken soup inhibit neutrophil (the major fraction of white blood cells) migration. Neutrophil activity can stimulate the release of mucus in the nasal cavity, which may be the cause of the coughs and stuffy nose caused by upper respiratory infections of cold viruses. Chicken soup could play a mild anti-inflammatory role that may perhaps lead to a temporary easing of the symptoms of illness. However, because of its weak efficacy, it cannot be used as the main method to cure the common cold.

## Vitamin C

Vitamin C was promoted as a cure for the common cold by a very famous scientist, Dr. Linus Carl Pauling, in the 1970s. Vitamin C, at high intake levels, has the effect of suppressing inflammation of the blood vessels. A clinical study showed that those who had the highest plasma vitamin C levels or took supplements of vitamin C had much lower levels of inflammatory markers in their bloodstream than those who did not.

The use of vitamin C in the prevention or treatment of the common cold and respiratory infections remains controversial, and research is ongoing. This indicates that the efficacy, if any, must be very weak; otherwise, it would not be a divisive approach to curing colds.

For cold prevention, more than thirty clinical trials including over ten thousand participants have examined the effects of taking daily vitamin C. Overall, no significant reduction in the risk of developing colds has been observed. In people who developed colds while taking vitamin C, no difference in the severity of symptoms has been seen overall, although a small, significant reduction in the duration of colds has been reported (approximately 10 percent in adults and 15 percent in children). For cold treatment, numerous studies have examined the effects of starting vitamin C after the onset of cold symptoms. So far, significant benefits have not been observed. However, inflammation is the body's weapon to fight against cold viruses. Inhibiting inflammation alone cannot effectively cure the common cold.

## Over-the-Counter Drugs

Acetaminophen is a common over-the-counter (OTC) anti-inflammatory drug; a popular brand of it is Tylenol. Acetaminophen works by blocking the production of prostaglandins in the body. Prostaglandins are a group of potent chemicals in the body for powering inflammatory reactions. They are released during infection and inflammatory events. When the body detects an infection or an inflammatory trigger, it releases substances called interleukins. Interleukins aid in the communication among these white blood cells and draw cells involved in the immune defense of the body to the site of the infection or injury. Acetaminophen inhibits the function of an enzyme called cyclooxygenase, which is critical in the production of prostaglandins. When this enzyme is inhibited, the level of prostaglandin falls, and the body returns to its baseline set point. Numerous patients with colds have taken acetaminophen to relieve the suffering from a cold.

Ibuprofen, found in Advil and Motrin, is also a strong inhibitor for prostaglandin production. Ibuprofen is also widely used for alleviating these symptoms of the common cold.

However, these OTC drugs cannot cure the common cold even though they are strong in anti-inflammation. Simply, these drugs are lack antiviral activity.

To cure the common cold, we must have a method or product that can kill or remove cold viruses in the disease area – the nose.

# 6. Weakly Inhibiting Viruses Cannot Cure Colds Quickly

It is common sense that the first task in curing a cold is to eliminate cold viruses. As discussed in the previous chapters, the trigger of the damaging inflammation reaction is the cold virus. Without viruses, there would be no need for the immune system to launch the defensive inflammation. There is no prescriptive antiviral drug to kill cold viruses at the time of this book's publishing in 2011. Several weak antiviral products are available, however.

**Curing Colds Was Not Easy**

As we mentioned earlier, more than two hundred different viruses can cause the common cold. In the past, it was not that easy to cure the common cold. You rarely catch the same virus twice; therefore, each viral infection runs its own course. Without a one-for-all antiviral therapy, you cannot be certain to cure or get rid of the cold quickly. Before the medical breakthrough was published in June 2011, for a cold, you had a number of weak options to fight cold viruses, such as to keep warm, sweat them out, and to inhale warm vapor in order to stop the growth of these cold viruses. Some other approaches, such as drinking lots of boiled ginger water, juices, herbal tea, or lemon juice, are not that effective. Using some of the immune boosters are helpful in prevention but not effective in treatment of a cold. The key question is: can any of these approaches eliminate cold viruses quickly? The simple answer is no; none of them can. All of these approaches have limited efficacy.

Therefore, it is a good idea to turn to your own body. When symptoms of a cold set in, your body has natural ways of taking the virus out of your system, such as coughing to expectorate mucus that contains a lot of viruses, or producing a rise in temperature, a fever, to fight the existing cold virus. Why not help your body do more so you can feel well enough to go to work or school? You need to know more in order to help your body effectively.

The main reason a common cold doesn't go away quickly is that you are re-infecting yourself through the upper respiratory tract, mainly the nose. The germs in your nasal cavity are multiplying at high speed. During the early days of the cold, your body can get rid of some of these viruses, but the remaining viruses replicate more. That's why you feel much sicker after day 1 of symptomatic infection. After a few days, your body has developed a more powerful antiviral immunity, and the speed of virus destruction is greater than virus growth, so gradually all viruses are eliminated, and you get a full recovery. You may wonder if there is any approach you can take to change this equation toward a faster recovery.

## Zinc

Zinc is an essential mineral that is naturally present in many foods and is available as a dietary supplement. Zinc is involved in numerous aspects of cellular metabolism. It is required for the catalytic activity of approximately one hundred enzymes, and it plays a role in immune function, protein synthesis, wound healing, DNA synthesis, and cell division. Zinc supports normal growth and development of a fetus during pregnancy, childhood, and adolescence, and is required for the proper sense of taste and smell. A daily intake of zinc is required to maintain a steady state because the body has no specialized zinc storage system. The Institute of Medicine of the National Academy of Sciences, and the Food and Drug Administration (FDA) provided a recommendation for people to take zinc to maintain optimal health. The normal upper level of daily intake is 15 milligrams for adults.

Because of the large number of people taking dietary supplements in varying amounts, including zinc, the tables of recommended daily allowances (RDA) by the Institute of Medicine of the National Academy of Sciences is now supplemented with a new value, "tolerable upper limit," the largest daily intake amount that is unlikely to cause harm. The concept of tolerable upper limit for vitamins and minerals is pertinent only for supplemental products, because toxic amounts of vitamins and minerals are not available from natural food sources. The "tolerable upper limit" for zinc is 40 milligrams per day. If the daily intake of zinc is over 40 milligrams, toxic effects could occur.

It is reported that zinc competes with rhinovirus to occupy viral receptors on the epithelial membranes of the nasal cavity (Eby 2010); hence zinc plays an inhibitory role to viral infection. Zinc is found in many cold lozenges and some over-the-counter drugs sold as cold remedies. Since zinc-containing products are used as medicine, you should know about its safety and efficacy.

In five studies that tested zinc in doses lower than 75 milligrams, no benefits were identified. When the daily intake of zinc was in extremely high doses, such as 75 milligrams and above, zinc lozenges had the ability to cut the length of colds significantly. However, doses of over 75 milligrams of zinc are five times over the FDA's recommended daily zinc intake and almost double the Institute of Medicine of the National Academy of Sciences' tolerable upper limit level. A number of the studies also found that taking the zinc lozenges came with various adverse side effects, such as nausea, a bad taste in the mouth, and upset stomach.

**Echinacea**

According to a national survey conducted in 2007, echinacea ranked third in herbal supplement use by adults and first in supplement use by children. Many people try herbal supplements containing echinacea to combat the common cold as its components have some antiviral activities. Many researchers have been investigating this widely used herb to see whether it is effective in preventing or treating colds. One study was performed by Dr. Shah et al. and published in the Lancet Infectious Diseases in 2007. This study showed that echinacea can shorten the cold duration by an average of 1.4 days. The National Center for Complementary and Alternative Medicine (NCCAM) is the lead agency for scientific research on the diverse medical and health-care systems, practices, and products not generally considered part of conventional medicine. Three NCCAM-funded studies that compared echinacea with placebo did not find a benefit.

In one study, published in the New England Journal of Medicine in 2005, researchers led by Dr. Turner at the

University of Virginia School of Medicine examined *Echinacea angustifolia* root extracts for effects against rhinovirus, the virus that causes the majority of common colds. The researchers compared three echinacea preparations in tincture form, each with different phytochemical properties. Participants were 399 healthy young adults. They received placebo or echinacea (300 milligrams three times daily), beginning seven days before exposure to rhinovirus. None of the echinacea preparations in this study reduced the rate of infection, severity of symptoms, or inflammation.

In another study, published in *Annals of Internal Medicine in 2002*, researchers led by Dr. Barrett, at the University of Wisconsin-Madison evaluated the effects of unrefined echinacea (capsules combining *E. angustifolia* root and *Echinacea purpurea* whole plant) on cold symptoms. Participants were 142 college students with early symptoms of a cold. They received placebo or echinacea (1 gram six times on the first day and then three times daily, for up to ten days). Echinacea did not reduce the severity or duration of symptoms in this study.

In a third study, published in the Journal of the American Medical Association in 2003, Dr. Taylor and researchers from the University of Washington Child Health Institute evaluated echinacea for efficacy and safety in children with upper respiratory tract infections. The preparation was a syrup containing dried, pressed *E. purpurea* juice from the above-ground parts of the plant. The 407 participants received either a placebo or echinacea (3.75 milliliters twice daily for children ages two to five; 5 milliliters twice daily for children ages six to eleven). Analysis of data from upper-respiratory tract infections in these children found that echinacea did not reduce the severity or duration of symptoms and was associated with increased risk of rash.

A report from SA Time on August 30, 2011, indicated that the herbal cold remedy echinacea works no better than sugar pills, according to a new study. http://www.iol.co.za/lifestyle/echinacea-no-better-than-a-sugar-pill-1.1127783. All participants in the study who were given tablets-placebo or not, found their symptoms improved faster than those who were given no treatment, as long as they believed that echinacea was effective. More than seven hundred people aged twelve to eighty, all suffering from a common cold, were split into separate groups. One group had no pills, another echinacea, and the third group took a placebo pill. Those taking pills of any kind had colds that were on average 0.16 to 0.69 days shorter than those without pills, who had colds that lasted an average of 8.4 days.

According to National Center for Complementary and Alternative Medicines, National Institutes of Health http://nccam.nih.gov/research/results/spotlight/051805.htm, these above studies show little benefit of echinacea as compared to a placebo, but other studies have shown that echinacea does provide some relief from symptoms. Overall, results of echinacea research have been mixed. Challenges associated with conducting this research include identifying the most effective parts of the echinacea plant, evaluating differences among echinacea species, and determining proper doses and preparations.

## A New Approach to Killing Virus-Infected Cells

In a paper published on July 27, 2011, in the journal *PLoS One*, researchers led by Dr. Rider at MIT tested their drug against fifteen viruses and found it was effective against all of them—including rhinoviruses that cause the common cold, H1N1 influenza, a stomach virus, the polio virus, dengue fever, and several other types of hemorrhagic fever.

The drug works by targeting specific cells that are infected by viruses. Theoretically, it should work against all viruses. The published results showed the new drug was safe in the laboratory. It is hoped that this unique drug will be fully developed soon so medical doctors will have an antiviral drug to cure the common cold and other viral infections. It will take at least a few more years to have a commercially available drug, however.

# 7. Removing Viruses and Inflammation to Cure Colds

In the previous chapters, it became clear that to treat the common cold, we must effectively eliminate viruses and reduce inflammation. Since with the common cold, also called viral rhinitis, the infection is mainly in the nasal cavity, we can take a practical approach to curing colds by focusing our efforts there. It is a dream come true to be able to cure your own cold with a sound and safe method. You can cure your colds quickly, when you know how.

Let's talk about nasal irrigation. Nasal irrigation, or nasal cleansing, refers to the rinsing of the nasal cavity with warm salty liquid. Generally, it is a safe and easy procedure. Nasal irrigation may improve breathing and enhance the senses of taste and smell if the right solution is used. Moreover, many people perform it as a precursor to yoga or meditation practice, which both rely heavily on deep breathing. Nasal irrigation has been used for treating colds, sinusitis, nasal allergy, and other respiratory tract disorders. Many physicians and scientists have conducted a variety of clinical studies, and generally support this hygiene practice as it has a numerous health benefits. These relevant study publications are listed in the Reference section to help in locating the original publications. In the text, the first author's name is provided so readers can easily find that publication by following the alphabetic order in the Reference section.

Specifically, a few clinical studies found that performing nasal irrigation is helpful in reducing the severity of a viral cold. Due to the fact that the previous generation of irrigation devices and solutions were used, the efficacy were not profound. In June 2011, a new breakthrough independent clinical study was published. This is very exciting as we now have a new therapy to cure the common cold.

## Performing Nasal Cleansing Cured the Cold Very Effectively

Yes, finally, there is a very effective way to cure the common cold! The breakthrough medical research in curing the common cold was completed by a group of medical doctors led by Dr. Huafei Ao and published in the *Journal of Infectious Diseases and Immunity* in June 2011. These doctors had patients with a common cold or influenza perform nasal cleansing with the NasalCare® Nasal Irrigation Kit three times a day. They reported profound efficacy. Their key findings are explained in the following sections.

## Performing Nasal Cleansing Dramatically Reduced the Cold's Duration

The group of doctors conducted a controlled, clinical, and laboratory-observer-blinded three-group comparison study. The study was approved by their hospital's ethics committee. The study participants were workers from a large company whose employees normally came to the study hospital for treatment, which made it easy to conduct all needed follow-up visits. All participants were first clinically diagnosed with a viral infection. Then, they were further tested for the influenza virus antigen. All participants completed their daily symptom diary. They all came back to the clinic to have the day 4 and day 8 clinical follow-up visits. All of them completed the study treatment assignment. Nasal irrigation was performed three times a day—in the morning, at midday, and in the evening (at about 7:00 a.m., 1:00 p.m., and 8:00 p.m.) by the patients in the nasal irrigation groups. Patients in the control (or comparison) group were treated with the hospital's standard of care. The main approach was to treat fever or relieve nasal congestion. The physician who performed the clinical evaluation was blind to the patient's study group assignment. Likewise, laboratory technicians were blind to the patient's group assignment.

Patients in the control group had more than eight days of cold disease. But for the patients who were in the treatment group using the NasalCare® Nasal Irrigation Kit, the cold duration was cut by three to six days. The median reduction of the durations of the colds was 4.5 days. In the other words, the patients with colds who performed nasal irrigation only had two to five days of the cold.

For influenza, the World Health Organization (WHO) recommends isolating new patients for fourteen days, since that is the normal duration of influenza. Patients with the flu in this clinical study had an average duration of 5.5 days. Performing nasal cleanse with the NasalCare® Nasal Irrigation Kit cut the duration by 8.5 days. That is why the physicians who work with infectious diseases are so pleased to see the results of this breakthrough medical research.

It is well known that the symptoms and signs of a cold/flu will usually become worse in the first few days. This is due to the fact that the virus accelerates its growth speed after initial penetration of your epithelial cells, and your immune system then proportionally adds more firepower to win the battle. After the battle reaches a peak, the immune response overtakes the virus, and the symptoms gradually subside to be completely resolved in about seven to fourteen days. In this study, the doctors did indeed observe that the patients in the control group had an increase in the severity of their diseases each day until day 4 or 5. But the patients in the nasal irrigation group had decreased symptoms on successive days. So, it is not a surprise that the doctors reported the cold disease duration was cut by 4.5 days.

It is such encouraging news that performing nasal irrigation is a new way of curing the cold and the flu. Certainly, using NasalCare® to perform nasal irrigation is much more effective than using zinc or echinacea.

## Performing Nasal Cleansing Reduced the Cold's Severity Significantly

In the same clinical study, medical investigators had all the patients record the severity of their symptoms of viral infection in their "disease diary." The average symptom severity scores for patients in each group were similar on the day 1 visit (baseline). After collecting all the patients' disease diaries during the day 4 and day 8 office visits, the investigators analyzed the data and concluded that the severity of cold symptoms of the patients in the control group worsened from day 1 to day 4. However, in those patients treated with NasalCare®, the severity lessened the day after they started nasal irrigation. For patients in the control group, their mean viral infection symptom scores slowly but steadily increased from day 1 to 4 and then gradually declined. At the end of the study (day 8), they still had at least one viral infection symptom.

In contrast, those patients who performed nasal irrigation three times a day, showed no worsening in symptoms after nasal cleansing, and furthermore, the severity of symptoms quickly decreased on each successive day. On day 3, the reduction of cold symptoms scores for patients in the nasal irrigation groups were much better than the control group. On day 4 and thereafter, the viral infection symptom scores for patients in the nasal irrigation groups had returned to normal, unlike the scores of those patients in the control group.

On the day 4 and day 8 office visits, a physician who did not know the patients' assignment groups conducted the medical examinations for each patient. The medical examination data were very similar to the data reported by these patients. The signs of viral infection were much less severe in the nasal irrigation groups than in the control group.

It is pretty logical; when the inflammatory factors were washed out along with cold viruses, both sides of the battlefield dramatically reduced their number of fighters, so both infection and inflammation were suppressed. Therefore, the severity of the viral infection was reduced. That's why using NasalCare® to perform nasal irrigation is more effective than taking zinc or echinacea.

## Performing Nasal Cleansing Removed Viruses from the Nasal Cavity

In this clinical study, medical investigators determined that cold/flu viruses could be removed by performing nasal irrigation three times a day. During baseline visit on day 1, the patients had not yet performed nasal irrigation. Their nasal secretions tested positive for the influenza viruses. After performing nasal irrigation three times a day for three days, all patients, who had previously tested influenza virus positive, had nasal secretions that were virus negative by the day 4 office visit. Clinically, these patients had basically recovered from the viral infection. During the next office visit on day 8, all those patients again tested negative for the virus in their nasal secretions, and all patients were clinically fully recovered.

Because the patients could not come to the clinic every day to test for viruses in their nasal secretions, there is a chance that these viruses were cleansed out even before the Day 4 office visit. This indicates that timely performing nasal irrigation with the NasalCare® Irrigation Kit in treating the non-complicated viral infection may have the similar efficacy to the well-known antiviral drugs oseltamivir or zanamivir, since both of the two anti-flu drugs can reduce the duration of influenza by more than one day. Either drug must be taken for five days, and some side effects were reported. Drug resistance of the flu viruses also occurs quickly.

Using NasalCare® to perform nasal irrigation will not generate drug resistance, and there are no noticeable adverse effects. The limitation of performing nasal irrigation is unable to treat the lower respiratory tract (lung) viral infection. For the treatment of any lung infection, you need a physician to help you. However, at the beginning of the viral infection, when you—and even your doctor—may not know exactly if you are suffering from either a cold or flu before a viral laboratory diagnosis, it is a good idea to start an effective nasal cleansing to remove these viruses out of your nasal cavities.

To better understand the results, the medical investigators also determined the concentration of the cold/flu virus receptors in the nasal secretions. These virus receptors are critical for the virus to be able to enter into the epithelial cells to grow (replicate). If these receptors become unavailable for the viruses, the newly released cold viruses then cannot attach to the epithelial cells in the nasal cavities, then the repeat infection by the cold viruses will be inhibited. The study reported that the concentrations of the virus receptors in the nasal secretions among all groups were very similar before the study treatment. However, after performing nasal irrigation, the concentrations of the virus receptors in the nasal secretion of the patients were significantly lower than those from patients in the control (comparison) group.

## Performing Nasal Cleansing Reduced Inflammation of the Nasal Cavity

During the same clinical study, the otolaryngologist observed the inflammation status of the nasal cavity of the patients with colds on the day 1, day 4, and day 8 office visits. The inflammation status was not different on day 1 among all the patients; this was before starting the treatments. The patients in the nasal irrigation group had a significantly lower inflammation status on day 4 and day 8 than those in the control (comparison) group.

As these authors pointed out, the possible mechanism by which nasal irrigation reduced the severity of nasal inflammation could be due to removing inflammatory mediators, such as histamines, prostaglandins, and leukotriens, contained in nasal mucus. These inflammatory mediators not only create a hostile environment for viral replication; they also cause nasal tissue damage.

Dr. Terence Davidson's group conducted a clinical study and published their findings in *The Laryngoscope* in 2000. They compared changes in inflammatory mediators in patients with perennial rhinitis treated with nasal hyperthermia or hypertonic nasal irrigation. They demonstrated that the greatest decline in histamine levels occurred in the group using hypertonic saline nasal irrigation, with declines in leukotriene C4 levels occurring exclusively in this irrigation group, and not in the hyperthermia group. Their literature review indicates that nasal irrigation is effective in decreasing symptoms of nasal disease. The mechanism by which this improvement is hypothesized to work as follows:

1) improving mucociliary function,

2) decreasing mucosal edema,

3) decreasing inflammatory mediators, and

4) mechanically cleansing the infected mucus.

All in all, this medical breakthrough study provides the strong evidence that an effective nasal cleansing is a new and effective therapy for common cold, since it can remove both viruses and inflammatory mediators from nasal cavities. After removing cold viruses and cleansed out inflammatory mediators, as a result, these symptoms of the common cold became less severe and disappear very quickly.

Finally, human society has a new method to cure the common cold safely and effectively!

# 8. Understanding Nasal Irrigation Products

There are many commercially available nasal irrigation products. As far as the authors are aware, NasalCare® Nasal Irrigation System is the only one which has been clinically studied and shown to shorten common cold duration by an average of 4.5 days when used three times a day. Although the other products have not been clinically studied, they may be useful for shortening your cold duration. This chapter is to point out the characteristics of these products without specifying any name brand. It is in your best interest to understand the differences among these nasal irrigation products and use the optimal product to recover from the common cold as soon as possible.

These many different kinds of nasal irrigation products can be grouped in several ways. Based on the force for driving the liquid into nasal cavities, these products are classified as nasal sprays, bulb syringes, neti pots, hand-pushed syringe irrigators, electric motor–driven nasal irrigators, and hand squeeze bottles.

## Nasal Sprays

Nasal saline sprays are often used as an alternative to saline irrigations because saline spray was often perceived to be equivalent to and better tolerated than irrigation. However, based on the clinical studies, they are not equivalent. Dr. Melissa Pynnonen and associates in the Department of Otolaryngology in the University of Michigan Health System compared the effectiveness of nasal saline spray and nasal saline irrigation. Their study examined the disease-specific quality-of-life change in a general population of patients with chronic nasal and sinus complaints. The study result was very convincing, finding that nasal irrigation performed with a volume of 8 ounces and delivered with the positive-pressure bottle are more effective than nasal saline sprays over an eight-week period for treatment of chronic nasal and sinus symptoms.

These patients were a community-based population with self-reported symptoms. The medical investigators suggested that these benefits derived from nasal irrigation with saline were likely due more to local effects, including decreased viscosity of nasal secretions, decreased edema of the nasal mucosa, and removal of debris, bacteria, allergens, and inflammatory mediators by the mechanical "lavage" action of saline irrigation. The greater efficacy of nasal irrigation over saline spray may be due to the greater volume, increased delivery pressure, and mechanical debridement achieved with irrigations. From this study, it is clear that nasal irrigation is more effective.

Normal intranasal saline spray seems to have no effect in treating the common cold. Dr. Chris Butler et al. from the Department of General Practice at the University of Wales College of Medicine reported on this topic in *The Lancet* in 2002. It is known that sodium cromoglicate inhibits the receptor for human rhinoviruses, the cold viruses.

They investigated whether intranasal cromoglicate could shorten the duration of a common cold. They randomly assigned 290 children diagnosed with suspected acute viral upper respiratory tract infections (the common cold) into two groups by their family doctors, and respectively treated with either intranasal 4 percent sodium cromoglicate spray or intranasal normal saline spray. Follow-up was by daily symptom diary for two weeks and by telephone. The Canadian Acute Respiratory Illness and Flu Scale (CARIFS) score was the primary outcome measure. Between the two groups, there was no difference in recovery rate over the first week, side effects, or the number of re-visits to their doctors. Nasal spray either with a normal saline or 4 percent sodium cromoglicate had no therapeutic effect in treating a cold. Likewise, nasal spray with hypertonic or normal saline nasal spray has no effect in treating the cold.

## The Bulb Syringe

The rubber bulb syringe has long been used to clear nasal cavities, particularly those of infants. Generally, you start by laying your child down with his or her chin tilted up slightly and squirting one or two drops of nasal saline into your child's nose to moisten and loosen up the mucus before suctioning it out.

When you try to remove the mucus from your baby's nose, you should first squeeze the air out of the bulb of the syringe to create a vacuum, then gently insert the rubber tip into one nostril. Slowly release the bulb to suction out mucus. Remove the syringe and squeeze the bulb forcefully to expel the mucus into a tissue or a container. Wipe the syringe and repeat the process for the other nostril. Of course, this procedure can be used by people of any age. However, for adults and anyone five years and above, there is a much better device than the bulb syringe.

This procedure is good for babies as there is no other simple method to suck the excessive mucus out from the baby's nose, but it does not actually irrigate the nasal cavities of adults. It is difficult to get an effective nasal cleansing this way.

**Neti Pots**

A neti pot holds the irrigating solution and gravity causes it to run into the nasal cavities. Neti pots are traditionally made of ceramic, plastic, glass, or metal. This simple device has been used for hundreds of years and is beneficial in promoting health in general, and reduced suffers from a variety of disorders. Many doctors, including Dr. Oz, recommend nasal irrigation with a neti pot. For those users who prefer using gravity for nasal irrigation, the neti pot is the choice. However, several new and better devices are available for nasal irrigation, and there are several concerns regarding the use of neti pots for treating the cold or flu.

Firstly, since all neti pots rely on gravity alone, the user has to tilt her or his head or turn it sideways in order to let the liquid run through the nasal cavity from the higher nostril to the lower nostril. Some users are unable to use the neti pot because of neck pain or shoulder stiffness.

Additionally, gravity exerts a limited force in irrigating sinuses. A scientific study conducted by Dr. Abadie et al. in 2011 shows that the neti pot can only let the liquid enter the lowest pair of sinuses, not the other sinuses at the higher positions.

The health concern is its potential risk of causing an infection in some users. As shared on the popular website eHow, one of the side effects of nasal irrigation with a neti pot is ear discomfort or pain. "The saline solution could also back up into the ear. This fluid in the ear could lead to infection." (http://www.ehow.com/about_5117560_side-effects-nasal-irrigation.html).

A long term use of a neti pot and its risk of infection was studied by Talal M. Nsouli, MD, clinical professor of pediatrics and allergy/immunology, who reported his study at the American College of Allergy, Asthma, & Immunology 2009 Annual Meeting. He found that "contrary to popular belief, irrigating the nose every day with the help of a neti pot may actually make patients more susceptible to sinus infections." http://www.medpagetoday.com/MeetingCoverage/ACAAI/16870.

Therefore, a neti pot, as an older device, is not an optimal choice of the nasal irrigation system. The authors do not recommend using a neti pot to treat the common cold or the flu at the current time since a newer and more advanced device is commercially available.

Furthermore, certain neti pots have a large opening and no lid. When the user pours liquid into one nostril, the liquid may leak out from the large opening onto the user's face. Even though some neti pots have a cover lid, if the lid is not tightly connected to the pot, it can fall off, or the liquid may leak out from the open-top onto the user's face, causing a problem.

## Hand-Push Syringe Irrigators

These are oversized syringes with nostril fittings. After you draw the solution from another container, you need one hand to hold the syringe body and one hand to push the solution run into your nasal cavity. Generally, this type of irrigator cannot hold a large volume of the irrigation solution. After completing each irrigation with a small volume of solution, you have to remove the nostril fitting before redrawing the solution from a large container. However, you need to irrigate your nasal cavity with a large volume in order to effectively remove viruses. Although this type of irrigator is not that user-friendly and you need another container in which to make the irrigation solution, you can largely avoid backwash contamination if you can keep pushing, not pulling, the syringe during the irrigation process. Another potential benefit is that you are performing nasal irrigation with a known volume of solution each time. However, its efficacy in treating a cold has yet to be clinically determined.

## Electric Motor–Driven Irrigators

Nasal irrigation machines that utilize electric motor–driven pumps have been available for about thirty years. These irrigation devices pump saltwater solution through a tube, in connection with a nasal adapter tip designed to seal against the nostril. Some of these machines have a few settings so you can choose the right liquid volume and/or speed. To do that, you adjust the dial to regulate pump speed and volume per minute.

Most of these motorized machines use a pulsatile or pulsating water pumping action at a relatively low, predetermined fixed pulse cyclic rate, designed to match the normal wave rate of a healthy, unobstructed nasal membrane surface (cilia). This matched pulse rate helps to stimulate the nasal cilia hairs and promote better sinus health, while reducing the severity of nasal inflammation. The more sophisticated motorized irrigators have two or more pulse cycle settings that adjust the actual pulse cycle. Some only have a simple volume/speed control, which does not alter the pulse cyclic rate. This design affords the user the option of using a higher pulse cyclic rate when suffering from partially closed sinuses, as in typical viral sinusitis. The efficacy of these motorized pump irrigators has not yet been compared to hand-squeezed nasal irrigators for treating cold or flu infections.

Generally, electric motor–driven pumps cost more, and if rechargeable, the battery quality is a concern. It is heavy and not convenient for travel. You may also unlike having the electric motor kept near the sink. In addition, cleaning the water tank and all parts after each use takes a good bit of effort. Nonetheless, it will not cause backwash contamination.

## Hand-Squeeze Nasal Irrigators

These are commonly known as squeezable bottles. This type of nasal irrigator introduces the liquid into the nasal cavities with positive pressure applied by the user's hand. The process of nasal irrigation provides a more complete rinsing without resorting to special techniques, such as holding the head to one side. These over-the-counter products are essentially bottles made of flexible plastic with a special tip to fit the nostril, or a nostril fitting. The nostril fitting also has a tube attached to it so that the irrigation solution can flow up into the nasal cavity. There are several types of squeeze bottles currently on the market; each has its own characteristics.

### *Squeeze Bottles without Valves*

This type of squeeze bottle has a few components: a soft bottle, a nostril fitting, a cap, and a tube to transfer liquid from the bottle through the nostril fitting into the nasal cavities. Some are ready-to-use, with the solution pre-filled. Additionally, some have a large volume, while others have a small volume. This kind of bottles have the advantage of simplicity, a lower cost for a single purchase for the bottle, and no need to tilt your head when performing nasal cleansing. However, several disadvantages exist:

1) Potential backwash contamination. Because there is no liquid valve, it is possible for the solution to flow back into the bottle after it has washed out the nasal cavity and sinuses.

2) Cannot continually irrigate. This kind of bottle has no air valve, so after you squeeze, liquid leaves causing negative pressure (a vacuum). Unless you let air come into the bottle, through the same opening the solution travels through, you cannot squeeze again. The negative pressure also encourages backwash (See Figure 8-1).

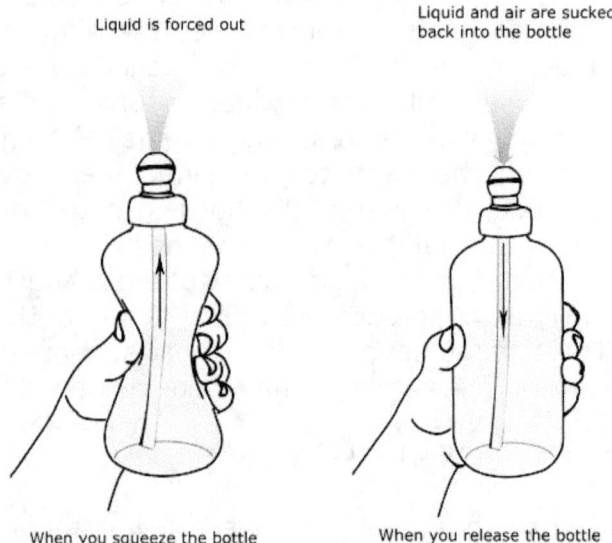

Liquid is forced out

Liquid and air are sucked back into the bottle

When you squeeze the bottle

When you release the bottle

Figure 8-1. What may happen if you use a squeeze bottle without valves

(2) Some of these irrigators hold 6 oz (180 ml) or less of irrigation solution. It is unknown if the reduced amount of irrigation solution could have the same treatment results presented earlier.

3) Time consuming. Due to the potential risk of backwash contamination, unless you throw it away after one use, you need to carefully clean the bottle, nostril fitting, and the tube. You may need to use a special disinfection solution and high temperature to sterilize the whole system after each use.

4) May cost more. You may need to buy this kind of bottle frequently. Medical doctors recommend that this kind of bottles need to be replaced every other week to avoid the potential problems (Welch et al, 2009).

5) Potential ear pressure. If the bottle is very soft and the diameter of the hole in the center of the nostril fitting is large, some users may easily generate a large wave of solution when the bottle is squeezed. The sudden force may cause ear pressure for some users.

**Irrigators with One Air Valve**

This type of squeeze bottle consists of a soft bottle, a nostril fitting, a tube to transfer liquid from the bottle through the nostril fitting into the nasal cavity, and a cap with an air valve. The advantage of this model is its simplicity, as only basically three parts require your attention during irrigation and maintenance, since the air valve is fixed into the cap (Figure 8-2). Certain disadvantages are listed below:

- The risk of backwash contamination still remains since there is no liquid valve, it is possible to have the contaminated solution flow back into the bottle.

- Although this model has an air valve, after you squeeze, the liquid and air compete to enter the bottle under the negative pressure. Obviously, liquid is heavier and enters the bottle before air. Therefore, having only one air valve cannot prevent backwash contamination (see Figure 8-2).

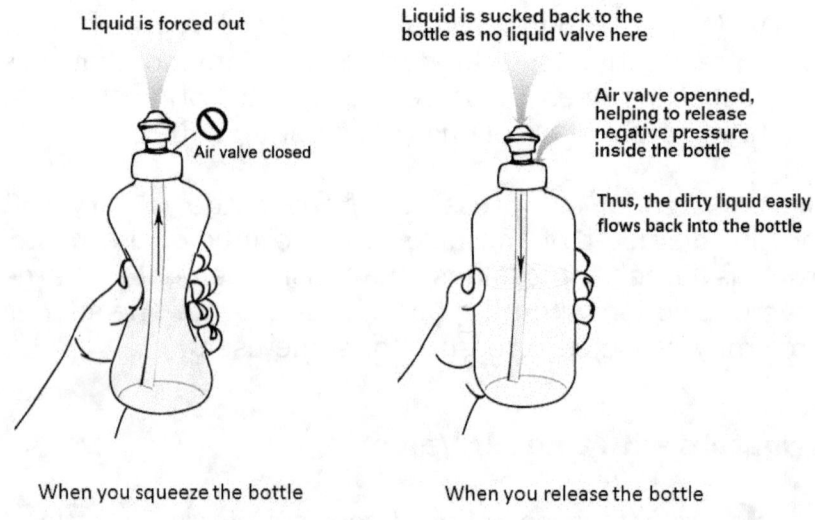

Liquid is forced out

Liquid is sucked back to the bottle as no liquid valve here

Air valve closed

Air valve openned, helping to release negative pressure inside the bottle

Thus, the dirty liquid easily flows back into the bottle

When you squeeze the bottle

When you release the bottle

Figure 8-2. What may happen if you use a squeeze bottle with one air valve

- you need to take many steps to clean the bottle and the thin tube due to the potential risk of backwash contamination.

- It is unsure if you can remove out these cold viruses from your nasal cavities effectively due to the potential contamination from the backflow fluid.

- May cost more. You may need to buy this kind of bottle frequently. Doctors recommend that the backflow prone bottles need to be replaced every other week to avoid the potential health problems.

### Irrigators with One Liquid Valve

This type of squeeze bottle has a soft bottle, a nostril fitting, a tube to transfer liquid from the bottle through the nostril fitting into the nasal cavity, and a cap with a liquid valve. As with the previous irrigators, the advantage of this model is its simplicity; again, only three parts need your attention during irrigation and maintenance, since the liquid valve is a part of the cap.

However, several disadvantages do exist: Although there is a liquid valve, it is not easy to have continual and effective irrigation. The bottle is full of negative pressure after your first squeeze (see Figure 8-3). You have to uncap it slightly to let air enter the bottle to balance the negative pressure before the next squeeze. This type of irrigator is not user-friendly and is time-consuming.

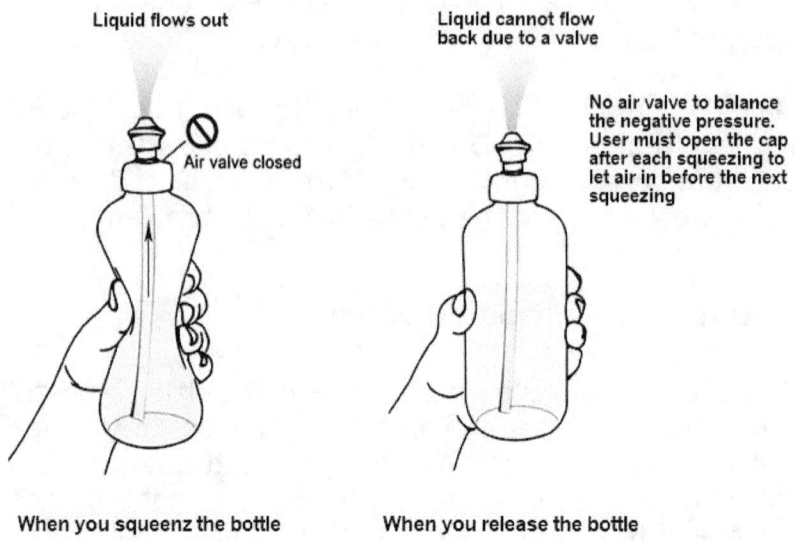

Liquid flows out

Air valve closed

When you squeenz the bottle

Liquid cannot flow
back due to a valve

No air valve to balance
the negative pressure.
User must open the cap
after each squeezing to
let air in before the next
squeezing

When you release the bottle

Figure 8-3. What may happen if you use a squeeze
bottle with one liquid valve

## Irrigators with Both Air and Liquid Valves

This type of squeeze bottle (Figure 8-4) is composed
of a soft bottle, a nostril fitting, a tube to transfer liquid
from the bottle through the nostril fitting into the nasal
cavity, the cap equipped with an air valve and a liquid
valve, and an "O" ring inside the cap. This model also has
the advantage of simplicity, as only four parts really need
your attention during irrigation and maintenance, as the
air and liquid valve are pre-assembled into the cap. The
liquid and air valves work in tandem, which means that
while one is open, the other is closed, to let you
continually generate a pulsatile liquid flow for nasal
irrigation.

The disadvantages of the above bottles are largely eliminated with this design. Why?

- Since there is a functional liquid valve, it prevents 99.6% of the contaminated solution from flowing back into the bottle according to the test results from an reputable independent laboratory (see Figure 8-4).Additionally, the air valve opens after you release the squeezed bottle, causing the negative pressure to disappear very quickly. You can continually irrigate your nasal cavities by repeatedly squeezing and releasing.

- You also have control over the pressure and volume of solution introduced by repeating the squeeze-release actions;

- This is the only one kind of squeeze bottle (patent protected) you can use to generate a pulsatile flow for nasal irrigation.

- The gentle flow of the liquid enables you to irrigate these sinuses and nasal passage without causing ear pressure.

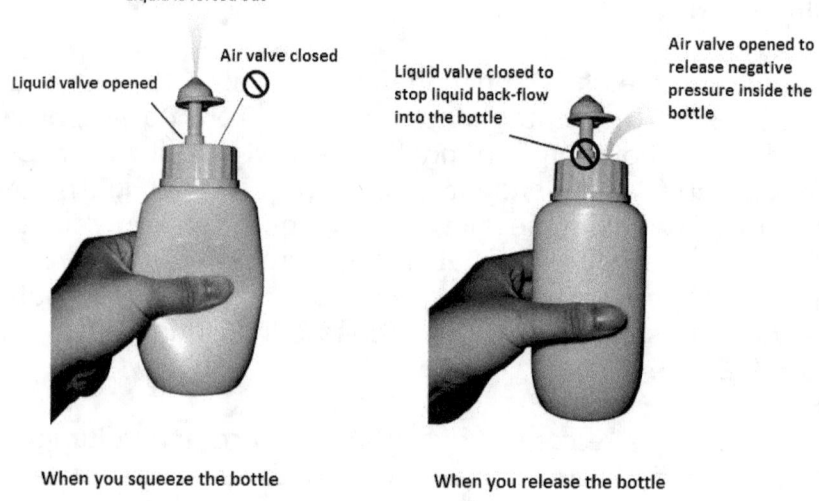

Figure 8-4. What may happen when you use a squeeze bottle with both liquid and air valves

A Canadian ENT group (Dr. Chang et al 2009) studied and concluded that "sinus irrigation bottles are a potential source of sinus re-infection. We recommend that patients change their irrigation bottles on a biweekly basis and clean them after each use. A sinus irrigation bottle without tubing and one that is not prone to nasal backflow may be an alternative option."

These comparisons and the doctors' recommendation indicate that you should use the nasal irrigator equipped with a functional anti-backwash valve system. The squeeze bottle must have both air and liquid valves to ensure a continual irrigation for safe and effective cleansing. The NasalCare® irrigator is the only one equipped with the two valves since its technology is patent-protected. As far as the authors are aware (up to this book's publishing), no other irrigators have been clinically shown to have such an effect.

## The Solution

Simply put, not all liquids are appropriate for nasal cleansing. Different solutions can change the structures and functions of nasal cavities. Therefore, it is important to discuss the following structures and functions of the components of the nasal cavity to understand how liquid choice affects them.

The mucous membranes, or mucosa, lining the nasal airways consist of two layers: the first layer is the luminal surface epithelium, and the second layer is the underlying connective tissue that supports and protects the surface epithelium. The latter layer contains various types and amounts of blood and lymphatic vessels, nerves, glands, and immune cells—they are embedded in the connective-tissue matrix. Most of the luminal surfaces of the nasal mucosa (with the exception of the most proximal regions of the nasal vestibule) are covered by a watery, sticky material called mucus. Its physical and biological properties are well suited for its role as an upper airway defense mechanism, filtering the inhaled air by trapping inhaled particles and certain gases or vapors.

Mucus is produced by mucous cells in the surface epithelium and sub-epithelial glands in the second layer. Once it traps foreign materials, such as dust or pollen, the cilia help move it to the nasopharynx, where it is then propelled into the esophagus and cleared in the stomach.

This upper airway apparatus is one of the first lines of defense against inhaled microbial pathogens, dusts, irritant gases, and toxicants. Therefore, any harmful materials that could induce compromises in nasal defense capabilities could also lead to increased nasal infections and increased susceptibility to lower respiratory tract diseases. Accordingly, the solution used for nasal irrigation must be biologically suitable to avoid any damage to the mucous membranes.

## Pure Water Is Not Suitable for Nasal Cleansing

Water is the most common liquid for body cleansing. However, water, no matter how sterilized, is not a good solution for nasal irrigation because the epithelial cells in your nasal cavity will experience toxicity if pure water is used. These living cells in your nasal cavity are healthy in the environment of the physiological liquid-like serum, which has an osmolality (a measure of the concentration of electrolytes)

The osmolality is the measurement of concentration of electrolytes in the liquid. The standard is the normal serum which has the normal range of 285 to 295 mOsm/liter. Here, mOsm is milliosmole; one thousandth $(10-3)$ of an osmole. The osmolality range of a physiological liquid can be a bit large, from 280 to 320 mOsm/liter. However, the osmolality of water is 0. This imbalance of electrolytes (no electrolytes) will damage the tissues and cells in your nasal cavity, opening your body to invasion by viral or bacterial pathogens. Therefore, you should never use pure water to irrigate your nasal cavities.

Dr. Michael Benninger published his research on this topic in the *American Journal of Rhinology* in 1994. He examined whether swimming pool water could hurt nasal function, as he observed that swimmers often complained of nasal dryness, and many had an increased incidence of chronic rhinosinusitis ("swimmer's sinusitis"). He compared the effect of swimming pool and ocean water on nasal mucociliary transport with a standard test and found that nasal mucociliary transport time was significantly prolonged after administration of swimming pool water, in comparison to ocean water under the same test conditions. As a hypertonic solution, the ocean water caused no harm to nasal function.

## Normal Saline Is Not Good for Nasal Cleansing

Normal saline contains 0.9 grams of sodium chloride per one liter of pure water. Its osmolality is 308 mOsm/liter. However, normal saline is not the optimal solution for nasal irrigation, since it only contains sodium chloride and is not pH balanced. Medical studies reported that using normal saline to irrigate the nose caused nasal dryness and other side effects, such as inhibition of nasal cilia movement. Nasal cilia movement is a natural way to detoxify environmental pollutants inhaled into the nasal cavity and must be maintained.

Dr. Melissa Pynnonen and colleagues at the University of Michigan Health System conducted a randomized controlled clinical trial in 2007. Their study observed certain adverse effects of using a normal saline (isotonic saline) solution, regardless of whether the normal saline was delivered by a squeeze bottle or by a nasal spray. In both groups, some patients had symptoms, such as dryness in the nose and pressure in the ears. Their results were similar to other published studies.

They also observed that subjects in the irrigation group were more likely to suffer these adverse effects than those in the nasal spray group. This randomized study did not find decreased medication use with the normal saline treatment.

## Nasal Saline Spray and Nasal Mucosa

Dr. Mark Boston and associates at the Children's Hospital Medical Center in Cincinnati performed a study in the laboratory and in human volunteers in 2003. They demonstrated that nasal saline spray containing a commonly used preservative agent (benzalkonium chloride), even at concentrations far lower than those in commercially available preparations, damaged respiratory mucosa, decreased mucociliary activity, and inhibited neutrophil (the major white blood cells) function in the laboratory tests. They also found that nasal saline spray was toxic to neutrophils in the human volunteers when applied to their oral mucosa. In comparison, these effects were not seen with phosphate-buffered saline.

The release of inflammatory mediators from lysed neutrophils into surrounding tissues may lead to the recruitment of other neutrophils and immune cells to the area. Therefore, it is possible that the lysis of mucosal surface neutrophils can result in a local inflammatory response in the absence of pathogenic microorganisms. Because nasal saline sprays are often used multiple times a day, the clinical significance of neutrophil cell lysis may be greater than that associated with nasal sprays used only once or twice a day.

## Buffered Normal Saline Is Not Optimal

Dr. Andrew Talbot led a group of researchers in conducting a clinical study, which was published in the Laryngoscope in 1997. For ten years, Dr. Talbot and other physicians had recommended buffered hypertonic saline (with a higher concentration of electrolytes than inside cells) nasal irrigation for patients with acute/chronic sinusitis and for those having undergone sinus surgery. To verify if their approach was right, they performed a study using healthy volunteers without any significant sinonasal disease. Patients served as their own comparison to test the nasal membrane transportation function. The "saccharin clearance test" was done before any nasal irrigation was performed. The volunteers then used one of two solutions to irrigate the nose, either buffered normal saline or buffered hypertonic saline. After they used one of the two solutions to perform nasal irrigation, a second saccharin clearance test was performed. On a separate day, the self-comparison test was repeated, followed by irrigation with the alternate solution and a second saccharin clearance test. The outcome of the study showed that nasal irrigation with the buffered hypertonic saline improved nasal mucociliary transportation function, while the buffered normal saline had no such effect.

## Buffered Hypertonic Saline Is Better

Doctors at Raleigh Ear, Nose, and Throat recommend their patients use warm saltwater as a preferred liquid for nasal irrigation (http://raleighent.com/). Simply, this solution is much more comfortable. The amount of salt added will depend on the patients' tolerance. Generally, the more salt that is added, the greater the decongestant affect. They also used bicarbonate which is a buffer (to maintain a balanced pH) to make the saltwater be less irritating.

There are several benefits of the buffered hypertonic saline for nasal irrigation. The hypertonic saline, like seawater, acts as a solvent and washes out mucus crusts and other debris from your nose. The higher salt concentration pulls fluid out of the swollen membranes and shrinks them. This decongests and improves the air flow into your nose. It helps sinus passages to open. A high concentration of saltwater and an alkaline irrigation (baking soda) improves nasal membrane cell function, such as nasal membrane transportation.

The solution made from dissolving a NasalCare® packet is a bicarbonate, citric acid, and sodium citrate buffered hypertonic solution. The salt is sea salt. It also contains an added moisturizing agent, aloe extract. Therefore, the NasalCare® buffered hypertonic solution of is ideal for nasal irrigation.

## Hypertonic Saline Nasal Spray on a Cold

Dr. Patricia Adam and associates conducted a study to determine whether hypertonic saline nasal spray relieves nasal symptoms and shortens illness duration in patients with the common cold or acute rhinosinusitis. Their study was published in 1998 in the journal *Archive of Family Medicine*. One hundred forty-three adult patients with a cold or sinus infection were randomly assigned to one of three groups:

1) Those treated with a hypertonic saline nasal spray three times a day;
2) Those treated with a normal saline spray three times a day;
3) Those who received no treatment.

The patients completed a 7-day symptom checklist that included a well-being question ("Do you feel back to normal?"). Nasal symptom scores (the sum of scores for nasal congestion, rhinorrhea, and headache) on day 3 and the day of well-being (the day of symptom resolution) were calculated. No difference was found in the cold duration among the three groups. That means that hypertonic saline nasal spray and normal saline nasal spray were no different as compared with no treatment at all. The investigators concluded that hypertonic saline does not improve nasal symptoms or illness duration in patients with the common cold or rhinosinusitis.

From this study, it is clear that nasal spray with either hypertonic saline or normal saline is not an effective cold therapy. The delivery method and the volume of the irrigation solution are very important.

## Home Made Nasal Irrigation Solutions

It is known that you can dissolve 1.8 grams of table salt in water to make 200 milliliter of solution, a normal saline. You can also dissolve a combination of 1/4 teaspoon of non-iodized table salt and 1/8 teaspoon of baking soda (optional) per 1 cup (8 ounces) of water. When it comes time to use the saline solution, the water temperature should be comfortably warm for you - not too cool and definitely not too hot, so be sure to test it first with your finger.

As you may know, some doctors suggest that their patients use hypertonic solutions (those with a higher salt concentration) for its better efficacy, while some other doctors recommend isotonic solutions. The simple explanation is that isotonic solution resembles the salt concentration of body fluids. The authors respect the results from these scientific studies: use the hypertonic solutions, but not overly hypertonic. Finding the right balance of salt is important because using too much tends to cause a burning sensation when using a nasal irrigation. Unless you have an analytical balance at home to weigh the salt or baking soda, you may not be able to make the solution to meet your need. To avoid the risk of losing your sense of smell, you can simply purchase the commercially available pre-mix, or refill, to make the irrigation solution.

To summarize the facts presented above, the choice of these solutions for performing nasal cleansing should be in the following order, from best to worst:

1) Hypertonic saline made with sea salt, buffered with sodium bicarbonate, citric acid, and sodium citrate with additional aloe extract.

2) Hypertonic saline made with table salt and buffered with sodium bicarbonate.

3) Isotonic saline made with table salt and buffered with sodium bicarbonate.

4) Isotonic saline made with table salt without any buffering agent.

Pure water should never be used for nasal irrigation.

# 9. The Advanced Nasal Cleanse System for Curing a Cold

The medical investigators used the advanced nasal irrigation system, NasalCare® Nasal Rinse Kit in a clinical study and observed a profound efficacy in curing common cold. This system won the Best New Product award during the 2010 US-Canada Efficient Collaborative Retail Market Conference for Cough & Cold and Allergy. We will do our best to present you what we know in this chapter. As the inventors of this system and trained scientists, we must fulfill our obligation to provide you the truth and facts, no more and no less.

## The Advanced Delivery Device

The nasal irrigator in the NasalCare® Kit has one-way air and liquid dual-valve technology, protected by two US patents (Liu 2001; Liu 2004; Liu and Zhang 2004; Liu and Zhang 2005). No other nasal irrigator has this unique feature. Figure 9-1 is a diagram of the NasalCare® Nasal Irrigator. After squeezing the bottle to pump the solution into the nasal cavity, you release your grip. At that moment, the liquid valve closes to stop backwash, and the air valve opens to let air flow into the bottle to balance the pressure inside the irrigator. When you repeatedly squeeze and release, you continually pump the solution with a moderate volume per squeeze into the nasal cavities to have an effective and continual nasal cleansing.

**Liquid flowing out**

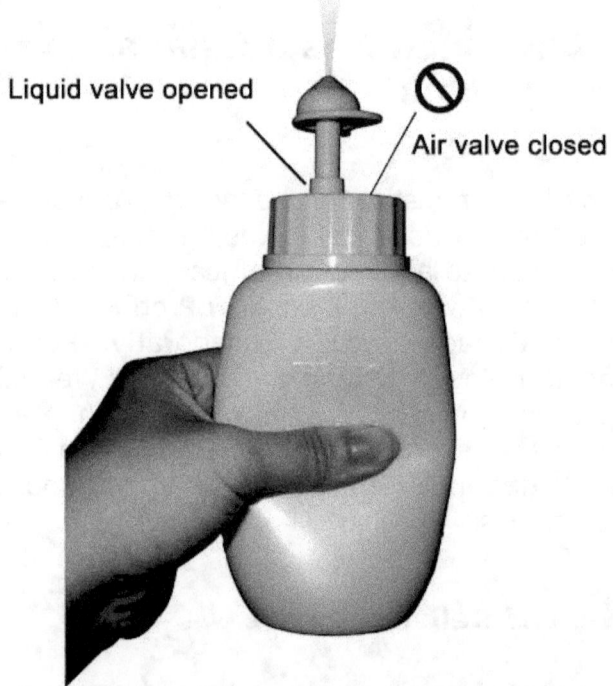

Liquid valve opened

Air valve closed

**When you squeeze the NasalCare Irrigator**

Figure 9-1. NasalCare®'s dual valve technology (when squeezed)

Many users have voluntarily provided testimonials that this nasal irrigator is much better than the neti pot. After trying this irrigator, they never used the neti pot again.

## The Advanced Nasal Irrigator Is Physically Safer Than the Bottle without Valves

The NasalCare® irrigator is physically safer than the nasal rinse bottles without any valves, or with only one air valve. When a bottle has only one air valve, the irrigator cannot stop backwash (see Chapter 8 for more details).

As determined by a nationally well-known independent laboratory, the NasalCare® irrigator eliminates 99.6% of backwash contamination, for a backwash rate of only 0.4%. On the other hand, for bottles without any valves or with only an air valve, the backwash rate is greater than 99%, as reported by the same independent laboratory.

## The Advanced Nasal Irrigator Continually Delivers a Clean Solution into the Nasal Cavity

The NasalCare® irrigator is also equipped with a one-way air valve. After you squeeze the bottle to pump the liquid into the nasal cavities and then release your grip, negative pressure is created within the bottle. While the liquid valve is closed, the air valve opens to let the air refill the space within the bottle (Figure 9-2). Then, you can squeeze again to pump the clean solution into the nasal cavity. Without this air valve, you would have to take the irrigator away from your nostril after the first squeeze and wait for the air entering the bottle to get rid of the negative pressure. Only after air enters can you squeeze the bottle again to get the solution into the nasal cavity, an added step that would greatly increase time spent on nasal irrigation. With the NasalCare® irrigator, the air and liquid valves work in tandem; the coordinated opening-closing actions of the two valves ensure that you have continual and pulsing nasal irrigation without interruption, which increases the efficacy of the nasal cleansing.

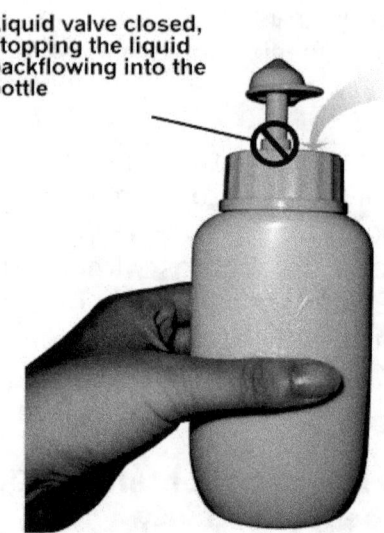

Liquid valve closed, stopping the liquid backflowing into the bottle

Air valve opened, helping to relaese negative pressure inside the bottle

When you release the NasalCare Irrigator

Figure 9-2. The Dual Valve System of NasalCare Irrigator (When released)

When you are trying to cure a cold, you don't want to have the cold viruses in the mucus flow back into the irrigator, letting any virus re-enter your nasal cavity to grow new viruses. For this reason, you should use the right nasal irrigator to do the nasal cleansing.

## The Advanced Nasal Irrigator Delivers the Right Amount of Liquid per Squeeze

Your nasal cavity has a limited amount of space; therefore, for nasal irrigation, the amount of solution sent from the irrigator into the nose should be moderate; you do not want to have a large amount in a very short time. As reported in the medical research published in 2007 by Dr. Bruce Turetsky et al. at the University of Pennsylvania, a normal adult male's nasal cavity volume for each side is about 7 milliliters (cc's), and a normal adult female's nasal volume is slightly less. It would be most comfortable if each squeeze of the nasal irrigator delivered about five (5) cc's, so the solution can gradually run through the nasal cavity.

The diameter of the central hole in the nostril fitting is one of the key factors for determining how much liquid runs through after each squeeze. If the diameter is too large and the bottle is very soft, one squeeze can deliver more than 50 milliliters of liquid from a 240 ml bottle, which is about seven times larger than the nasal volume. Having this much liquid under the high pressure could force the liquid to run into the wrong place, such as ears. As a result, this kind of bottle may cause ear pressure. For the NasalCare® irrigator, the diameter of the hole in the nostril fitting is 3 millimeters, which would allow about 4 to 6 milliliters (cc) to enter the nasal cavity per squeeze. It is recommended that you repeat the squeezing-releasing action two times per second. You will feel the liquid running into your nasal cavity gently and gradually, but slightly more forcefully than a neti pot in delivering the liquid.

A scientific study published by Dr. Abadie and collaegues in 2011 shows that NasalCare® can deliver solution to the three pairs of sinuses, while the neti pot only delivers the liquid into the lowest pair of sinuses. Unlike with the neti pot, when you use the NasalCare® nasal irrigator, you don't need to tilt your head, so you perform a neat, more effective and comfortable nasal irrigation.

## The Advanced Nasal Irrigator Is User-Friendly

Since the NasalCare® irrigator has more features than other squeeze bottles, you may wonder if it is still easy to use. Actually, using the NasalCare® irrigator is even easier than using some other nasal irrigation products, like a neti pot. There are just a few simple steps:

1) Uncap the irrigator;
2) Add the solution mix and warm water into the bottle;
3) Recap it and shake to dissolve the mix;
4) Insert the irrigator tip into your nostril;
5) Repeat the squeezing-releasing action;
6) Rinse the inside and outside of the irrigator with tap water, and let it air dry for the next use.

The opening of the NasalCare® bottle is wider than some other bottles, which allows you to add the formulated solution mix and water into the bottle easily and accurately. If the bottle opening of the irrigator is very small, you chance losing some of the mix, which will make the solution hypotonic, rather than isotonic, which may harm the sensitive nasal cavity. Many seniors and young children have a hard time holding a bottle steady for filling. The wider opening of the bottle of the NasalCare® irrigator will help make it easier to pour the refill mix and water into the bottle. The attention-to-detail design makes the NasalCare® irrigator truly user-friendly.

## Using the Advanced Nasal Irrigator Saves Time

The NasalCare® irrigator is very easy to maintain and to clean after each use. Because of its patent-protected anti-backwash technology, backwash contamination is essentially eliminated, as noted earlier. After each nasal irrigation, you can simply add tap water into the irrigator, shake it, and pump the water out. This leaves the tube, liquid valve, and the bottle free from salt accumulation. You can use a little brush and soap to clean the cap and nostril fitting, and then rinse them with tap water. Unless you use the irrigator for post-nasal-surgery cleansing or following your physician's special instructions, it is unnecessary to sterilize the irrigator after each use. It takes about one minute to clean the entire NasalCare® irrigator after each use with a liquid soap and water. For some other irrigators, you would have to spend much longer time to clean the tube and the bottle because of the risk of backwash contamination.

## Using the Advanced Irrigator While Traveling

The NasalCare® irrigator also has a protective cover. It prevents bacteria and debris from entering the irrigator. When you travel to a new place, you may come into contact with people who might be carrying cold viruses to which you have no immunity. Particularly, if you are attending a large meeting during the cold season, you will encounter people coming from many different areas, some of whom will be carrying their unique cold viruses. For your benefit, it is a good idea to perform nasal cleansing each night.

## Using the Optimal Solution to Cure Common Cold

As noted earlier, for nasal cleansing, the solution must be biologically friendly to the lining of the nasal passages and cavities. The last thing you want to do is to damage your nasal structure and function and impair your sense of smell. Therefore, it is critically important to use the optimal solution for performing nasal irrigation.

The solution made by dissolving the NasalCare® mix into 8 ounces (240 milliliters) of water is nasal-membrane friendly. Its ingredients are sea salt, aloe vera extract, sodium bicarbonate, citric acid, and sodium citrate. These ingredients are the best in their class. The solution is much better than buffered saline or non-buffered normal saline. These individual ingredients are reviewed below.

**Sea Salt**

Sea salt is produced by evaporating seawater, usually with little processing, which leaves behind some trace minerals and elements depending on the seawater source. These minerals add flavor and color to sea salt. Table salt, on the other hand, is mined from underground salt deposits. It is more heavily processed to eliminate trace minerals and usually contains an additive to prevent clumping. The flavor of sea salt is slightly less pronounced than that of table salt because of the lack of these additives.

It is also known that taking a sea salt bath can help reduce the risk of infection. Bathing in sea salt water can also serve as a pain reliever. The sea salt promotes the cells exchanging minerals with the water and then releases toxins from the body to improve the health of the patients. As a result, many users prefer the NasalCare® mix especially because of the sea salt.

**Aloe Vera**

Aloe vera extract has numerous health effects. Many scientific research papers have been published on the health benefits of aloe. The three main categories of effects of aloe are anti-inflammatory, antibacterial, and antiviral. Some research evidence indicates that aloe vera extract may be useful in the treatment of wounds, burns, minor skin infections, sebaceous cysts, diabetes, and elevated blood lipids in humans. These positive effects are thought to be due to the presence of certain compounds, such as polysaccharides, mannans, anthraquinones, and lectins. Aloe extract has been widely used in the cosmetic and alternative medicine fields because of its soothing, moisturizing, and healing properties. Aloe vera gel is used as an ingredient in commercially available lotions, yogurt, beverages, and some desserts. Aloe juice is said to be one of the finest body cleansers, cleaning morbid matter out from the stomach, liver, kidneys, spleen, and bladder and is also considered to be an effective colon cleanser. Aloe vera at an appropriate amount makes it a particularly beneficial ingredient in the NasalCare® solution mix.

## Sodium Bicarbonate

Baking soda is the more common name of sodium bicarbonate. One of the most important medical benefits of having sodium bicarbonate in the body is that it helps balance your blood acidity, or pH. If your blood becomes too acidic, bicarbonate can react with some of the excess acid and neutralize it. The act of breathing affects your blood pH, since carbon dioxide is acidic. Having bicarbonate in the bloodstream prevents your breathing from changing your pH. To this same end, sodium bicarbonate is one of the ingredients commonly used in hemodialysis, helping to regulate and maintain the pH of the blood.

Because of its safety and efficacy in body cleansing, sodium bicarbonate is a natural choice for including it in the NasalCare® Irrigation Refill Mix.

## The Citric Acid / Sodium Citrate Buffer System

Citric acid is an organic acid produced in nature, and it is a natural preservative. Sodium citrate is its salt. Found in citrus fruits, citric acid has hundreds of uses in medicine, in the food industry, in science, and in heavy industry.

For body cleansing, citric acid has the ability to bind with metals; that is, it can create bonds between binding sites at the molecular level.

Furthermore, a clinical study conducted by Dr. Panagiotopoulos et al. reported that introducing a citric acid and sodium citrate buffer improved the senses of smell. The study was done with patients who complained of a loss of the sense of smell. Using the citric/sodium citrate buffer, doctors significantly improved their patients' smell function.

The nasal cleansing solution made by dissolving the NasalCare® mix is a buffered hypertonic saline. It is comfortable, does not cause water toxicity, promotes the detoxification function of nasal cilia membrane without stinging, burning, or nasal discomfort, adds soothing and moisturizing elements, helps to prevent nose dryness and bleeds, is free of preservatives, and is clinically shown to enhance the sense of smell. In part because of this superior mix, the professional buyers for well-known national drug chain stores and retail chain stores voted overwhelmingly that the NasalCare Nasal Irrigation Kit was the "Best New Product" during the 2010 Efficient

Collaborative Retail Marketing Conference for Cough and Cold and Allergy. The NasalCare® Nasal Irrigation Kit is publicly recognized because of its unique and advanced irrigator and solution mix.

# 10. How to Cure a Cold in Two Days

It is achievable! Of course, it's not that easy to cure a cold in one or two day, but it is possible if you do it right. The popular Web site www.eHow.com provides a seven-step path to getting rid of a cold in a day. For comparison purposes, these seven steps are directly quoted below: (http://www.ehow.com/how_4494158_get-rid-cold-day.html):

1) Treat your symptoms immediately. When symptoms of cold set in, it is actually your body's way of taking the virus off your system, such as coughing to expectorate mucus, or fever to fight the existing cold virus. However, if you really need to feel well for the sake of your work or school, then treat your symptoms immediately. For nasal congestion you can treat it by either taking an oral decongestant or nasal spray. You can take cough suppressants if you have dry cough or cough expectorants if you have a productive cough (cough with phlegm). If you have fever associated with body aches, taking acetaminophen (such as Tylenol) will help ease your discomfort. Take lozenges to ease your throat.

2) Keep yourself warm and be properly rested. Bed rest under a warm blanket is the best way to assist your body while it's battling against the cold viruses in your system. It is normal for you to feel weak and drowsy when you're ill, so just stay relaxed and allow your body

to recover. The more you rest, the faster you heal. Take it easy if you want to get well sooner.

3)　Drink lots of fluid. Flush those cold viruses away by constantly drinking plenty of water. You can also go for flavored liquids such as warm lemon juice with honey, orange juice and other fruit juices. Chicken broth is very effective in reducing the activity of white blood cells (neutrophils) that can induce an increase in mucus production.

4)　Clear off that runny mucus. Blowing your nose more often is [more] advisable than sniffing it back to your nose. The more you blow it out, the more you take a part of the virus out of your system, but this has to be done in a correct way. Blow one side of your nose at a time. Press one nostril and gradually blow on the other side and then vice versa. Do not blow both your nostrils at once, for it may only create pressure that can lead to ear ache.

5)　Unclog that stuffy nose. You can do this by simply rubbing Vicks VapoRub on your back, chest, above your nose, and the space between your nostrils and upper lip. You can also massage the bridge of your nose with an up and down stroke using your index finger and thumb. The vapor of the menthol rub and the nose bridge massage will loosen up your obstructed nose and will help you breathe more easily.

6)　Eradicate that cold virus with steam inhalation. Boil 3 cups of water in a kettle. Prepare a bath towel, a medium-sized basin, and Vicks VapoRub. Position the basin into a chair and table where you can easily sit and do the steam inhalation process. Pour the boiled water into the basin, add a teaspoon of Vicks on it and mix. Then sit down and position your head above the basin, and cloak or surround the basin with your towel, allowing no steam to escape. Breathe in on the steam to relieve your stuffy nose and also to eliminate the existing cold virus (these type of viruses do not have the ability to survive at elevated temperatures).

7)   Soothe that scratchy throat. Mix a teaspoon full of salt in a mug of warm water and gargle. This will help ease your irritated throat. Do this gargling procedure 4 times a day. You can also relieve your cold-infected throat by sipping hot liquid. This is quite a challenging method because here, you are to sip the hottest water temperature you can handle. You can either use plain water or tea mixed with lemon. After sipping one mug of hot liquid, drink a small glass of pure water at room temperature. This hot water method will not only help ease your irritated throat but will also help in eliminating your cold virus quickly.

These seven steps, presented in the popular website, may or may not have the clinical studies to support.  And the authors are unaware of the new breakthrough clinical study. Nevertheless, it is good to know there are some approaches for you to take to cure a cold fast.

As you can see, the last two steps aim to eliminate cold viruses with hot water in your mouth or with evaporated water inhaled into your nose. This may be useful, but they are very weak methods of eliminating cold viruses. Even if you followed all seven of these steps, you might not get rid of a cold in one day.

But with NasalCare®, now you have a new way to get rid of the common cold possibly in one or two days.

## An effective Method to Cure a Common Cold Fast

Here is an effective approach to cleanse out cold viruses and inflammatory mediators immediately after you have the first symptom of the common cold: Whenever you started to have the common cold symptoms, you can perform an effective nasal cleansing with the NasalCare® Nasal Irrigation Kit every four hours during the day. Suggested times could be 8 a.m., 12 p.m., 4 p.m., and 8 p.m., or four hours after the previous nasal irrigation. The doctors who conducted the clinical study (Dr. Ao 2011) let the patients perform nasal cleansing in the morning, noon and evening, three times a day. You can do it either three or four times a day. Make sure the full eight ounces (240 ml) of liquid runs through your nasal cavities at each nasal cleansing.

Your symptoms might be gone by the next day since most viruses and inflammatory mediators can be removed from your nasal cavities after three or four times of nasal cleansing. Cold viruses cannot grow very fast if you perform nasal cleansing every four hours. Essentially, you eliminate the seeds for growing any new viruses. No virus growth means your body's immune system will have no need to send more white blood cells and inflammatory mediators to your nasal cavities to fight. This in turn decreases inflammation. Then, the cold symptoms are subsided or gone quickly.

Even if you feel like you have completely recovered from the cold, it is important for you to continue this simple nasal cleansing procedure for a few more days to make sure the viruses do not grow to cause a new symptomatic infection.

## Better Late than Never

If you did not perform an effective nasal cleansing soon after having the early symptoms of the cold, you will be unlikely to cure a cold very quickly. However, you should still start this procedure as soon as you can. If you repeat this practice every four hours, any newly released viruses and inflammatory factors will be effectively removed.

In the past, people were in the dark about how to cure the common cold, because there was no drug to kill these cold viruses, and the nasal cleansing process to remove viruses and inflammatory factors was unknown. Now you know how, and it is not hard to get it done. Timing is key, though. As an analogy, imagine a fire has just started in a very small area of a forest. It is easy to extinguish it quickly if the firefighters are there to act at the earliest possible time. When the fire becomes very large, it will take a much longer time to kill it. The same is true for treating your common cold, a viral fire in your nose.

However, if you do not remove these cold viruses, some bacteria will have a higher chance to infect you after the virus has damaged the lining of your nasal cavities.

## It Is a Numbers Game

You can have cold viruses in your nasal cavity without experiencing cold symptoms. The symptomatic infection caused by cold viruses is a numbers game. If only a few viruses are in your nose right now, the body's immunity will not launch a severe attack. Only when the cold viruses grow significantly in number will the immune system be alerted to start the fight. Only after the immunity starts the fight will the common cold symptoms show up. Your nose then becomes a battlefield for the war of the viruses against your immune system.

So how many viruses in your nose does it take to cause a symptomatic infection? This is a rather difficult question to answer. As you can understand, each person's health, nutritional status, stress level, immune system, contact with outside society, and so on are different. For medical research, scientists use the special unit, 50 percent tissue culture infectious dose ($TCID_{50}$) to determine how many infectious particles are in your nasal secretions. It is the quantity of the virus that will produce a cytopathic (cell damaging change) effect in 50 percent of the tissue cultures inoculated.

Let's put out a practical number here: if you have less than 100 $TCID_{50}$ of viruses in your nose, you would be unlikely to have any cold symptoms. If 10,000 $TCID_{50}$ viruses were there, your body's immune system would be able to detect it, and it would be a symptomatic infection. If not treated, these viruses, within hours or days, could replicate to 100,000 $TCID_{50}$. Your immune system then launches a dramatic inflammatory defense. Then, severe cold symptoms begin.

We hope that you will decide to perform an effective nasal irrigation to win the numbers game. Using the NasalCare® Nasal Irrigation Kit, you can largely remove these viruses from your nasal cavity. As a result, no further severe symptoms will develop. After you repeat this effective nasal cleansing a few more times, virtually all viruses could be removed. When that happens, your immune system has no further need to release these white blood cells and inflammatory mediators in the nose to kill the viruses.

In October 2010, I (James Liu) cured myself of a common cold in one day. On the first day after I returned home from a national scientific meeting held in Boston, I felt clearly that I had cold symptoms at about 3 p.m. I performed a nasal cleansing with the NasalCare® Irrigation Kit at that time and then repeated the deep nasal cleansing again at 7 p.m. and 11 p.m. I had a good night's sleep, and on the next day, I did not feel as if anything was wrong.

I made the same observation in 2010 with my son, who was a high school student at the time. One afternoon, he came home after tennis practice, and I heard him coughing and sneezing. When I asked what was going on, he told me that he was going to do a nasal irrigation. Since he had a NasalCare® Irrigation Kit in his bathroom, there was no need for me to say any more, other than to remind him to repeat the procedure about every three to four hours. He did. The next day, he drove himself to take the national ACT exam in the morning. On that same afternoon, he returned to the tennis courts. When I asked him where his cold was. He just said, "All gone."

You may wonder if this quick recovery can be achieved by others. As reported in the *Journal of Infectious Diseases and Immunity* in June 2011, a group of patients with common colds or flu used the NasalCare® Irrigation Kit to treat their viral infection. The majority of them reduced the severity of their cold symptoms in one day after performing an effective nasal cleansing. After two days of treatment with NasalCare® three times a day, their cold symptoms were significantly less severe than those of the patients in the control (comparison) group.

Could these patients do better? We think so. They all started using the NasalCare® Irrigation Kit after they were diagnosed by the physician, which was after they were already sick for one or two days. They therefore did not start the therapy as quickly as they could have. But if they had started the nasal cleansing within twelve hours of their first symptom, they could have recovered much more quickly.

It is hard to guarantee that you can cure your cold in one or two days. However, if you have a NasalCare® Irrigation Kit on hand when you experience the first cold symptoms and you immediately start to perform an effective nasal cleansing, you do have a high chance of curing your cold in one or two days. Your symptoms, if there are any left, might be mild enough that you can go to work or school without much concern. You can bring a NasalCare® irrigator and a few solution packets to work or school with you to continue your therapy. Since your nasal cavities will be largely cleansed, you will not have many virus particles to spread around. If untreated, you cough and sneeze in your office, making it very likely that you may infect others. The same is true at home with your family members.

More Effective than the Gold Lab Procedure in Removing Viruses scientifically formulated solution, you can remove about fifteen times (15X) more viruses than a clinical gold standard diagnostic procedure—namely, collecting nasal secretion specimens through a "nasal wash" with saline. Let's compare.

As you may hear, respiratory virus diagnosis depends on the collection of high-quality specimens. Virus is best detected in specimens containing infected cells and secretions. The World Health Organization (WHO) and the U.S. Center for Disease Control and Prevention (CDC) commonly recommend using a "nasal wash" to collect specimens for diagnosis of viral respiratory tract infections. Among these common methods of collecting specimens, including nasopharyngeal aspirate, nasal swab, throat swab, and nasopharyngeal swab, nasal wash is generally more reliable and more sensitive. It is the gold standard. Here is how to collect a nasal-wash specimen:

The patient sits in a comfortable position with the head tilted slightly backward. The patient is advised to keep the pharynx closed by saying "K" while the washing fluid (usually normal saline) is applied to the nostril by a medical professional, such as a nurse. With a transfer pipette, 1.0 to 1.5 milliliters of washing fluid is instilled in one nostril at a time. The patient then tilts his or her head forward and lets the washing fluid flow into a specimen cup or a Petri dish. The process is repeated with the alternate nostril until a total of 10 to 15 milliliters of washing fluid has been used. Depending on what type of virus is there, the quantity of the virus can vary from a few $TCID_{50}$ to $10^5$ $TCID_{50}$ in 1 milliliter of the washing fluid. A simple mathematical calculation is that this procedure can remove about one million virus units.

This nasal-wash procedure has been practiced by medical investigators for more than fifty (50) years. It must be true that the washing fluid has detectable viruses. You see the specimen is from the 10 to 15 milliliter solution. When you use 240 milliliters of NasalCare solution to perform an effective nasal cleansing when you have a cold, think how many more viruses can you remove under positive pressure. Sure enough, your way is much more effective than the WHO/CDC recommended procedure in terms of removing viruses. Therefore, you can have a high level of confidence now in the reasons why you should perform an effective nasal cleansing to cure a cold. Very quickly, you can win the numbers game.

Very simply, fewer viruses means less severity in the cold disease. No virus means no cold.

Although cold viruses can duplicate and release very quickly, they cannot match your removal speed when you perform nasal irrigation with 240 milliliters of solution every four to six hours.

If you'd like to recover faster, you can perform nasal cleansing with NasalCare solution every two hours. The solution is safe enough for frequent use during cold therapy. You don't give cold viruses a chance to grow. The cold viruses will lack seeds—since these viral seeds were cleansed out by your frequent nasal irrigation. You needn't worry about washing out those immune factors. They are called to fight against cold viruses. When the cold viruses are cleansed away, the immune factors will become unnecessary. In addition, these nonspecific immune fighters will not cause any further inflammatory reactions.

By performing a frequent nasal cleansing, you don't allow any fighters in your nasal cavity to launch any further attacks. Your cold symptoms will be gone when these bad and good fighters are removed.

## How to Start Nasal Cleansing Sooner

You know the cold symptoms. When you first feel the symptoms, you should start the nasal cleansing process with the NasalCare Nasal Irrigation Kit right away. The best practice is to keep one kit at home and one in the office even when you are not sick. As analogy, if you planned to go camping in the wilderness, you would bring a gun with you. It would be too risky not to, and it would be too late to buy a gun when you are approached by a big wild animal. If you have a family, this is even more important. Who knows which family member might catch a cold the earliest? If the NasalCare Kit is already there, the one who is sick can start the therapy without losing any time.

Everyone knows that to extinguish a fire, the most efficient way to fight is to start early. There's no need to wait until the fire becomes huge. A little fire can only cause a little damage, but a big fire causes a lot of damage. It is the same thing when you fight against a cold virus infection. It is probable that all your family members will catch a cold during the winter. It is the best practice for the family to have a NasalCare Kit there just in case.

## Where You Can Get a NasalCare® Kit

NasalCare® is sold over-the-counter at stores like Big-Y Foods, Bruno's Great Foods, Chamberlin's Natural Foods, Fruth Pharmacy, Giant Foods, Good Neighbor Pharmacy, Harmon Stores, Harris Teeter, Kimberton Whole Foods, Major Value, Medicap Pharmacy, Medicine Shoppe, Piggly Wiggly, SaveMart, Smith Drug, Southern Family Markets, Weis Market, and online stores, like www.amazon.com, www.cvs.com, www.drugstores.com, and www.hardtofindbrands.com. You may also be able to find NasalCare® at your local pharmacy; call ahead of time to verify.

You can also get the NasalCare® Nasal Irrigation Kit from the manufacturer by calling toll free 1-888-658-8108, or at the manufacturer's online store: www.nasalcleanse.com.

## Time Is on Your Side

During a viral cold, you can start nasal cleansing any time. The earlier you start, the quicker these viruses will be removed, and the earlier you can recover. Now you know it is critical to start the nasal cleansing as early as you can so you don't give cold viruses enough time to grow into a large quantity. If you start early, then your body's immune system will have no need to launch a severe attack against the cold viruses. That means the inflammation in your nasal cavity will be at a minimum. Thus, the symptoms and signs will be very mild — mild enough that they will not bother you as you continue to go to work or school.

## You Can Even Do Better—No Cold at All

You've just attended a big party where you met many people and you might have come into close contact with someone carrying cold viruses even though she or he did not show any cold symptoms. If someone is coughing or sneezing (previously shown in Chapter 2, Figure 2-2), you have a high risk to inhale these tiny aerosols in the air.

Having read this book, you know it is very beneficial for you to use the NasalCare system to perform a nasal cleansing after you come home. Those freshly inhaled cold viruses will be washed away before they even have a chance to enter the epithelial cells of your nasal cavity. Yes, please do yourself a big favor, since there is no fun in having a cold.

## Know Your Risks before Catching a Cold

If you are working in a cubicle and your co-worker next to you coughs and sneezes a lot during the non-allergy season, you have a good chance of inhaling cold viruses. If you are sitting in an airplane and a person sitting nearby you coughs and sneezes repeatedly, you have a high chance of inhaling some viruses. Before you read this book, you would have let the natural infection control you. Now, you can proactively control the event by using NasalCare to get rid of cold viruses you inhaled today. This way, you can prevent a cold or flu altogether.

## Day-Care Center Staff

It is easy to see how an infection spreads, especially in day-care centers. Children in day-care centers give infections to each other. They drool, and their noses drip. They touch each other and touch all the shared toys. This spreads infections. Although staff members of day-care centers are adults, they are constantly in contact with the children. These children carry all kinds of viruses, and the teachers are not immune to this many viruses. That's why they catch so many infections during a year.

Now you can protect yourself. When you notice a number of kids are sneezing and coughing and you cannot help inhaling viruses, you can perform nasal cleansing when you get home. Cold/flu symptoms generally appear two to three days later after the virus was inhaled. If you take the window of opportunity to perform an effective nasal cleansing, you can be free from the repeated infection.

The cold/flu viruses spread easily. What happens in a day-care center can also strike a community all at once. You should use NasalCare to perform nasal cleansing every day, so you will not help to spread these viruses around.

## Flight Attendants

You know that within an airplanes, passengers come from everywhere.  They potentially carry any kinds of cold viruses. In the sealed space, it is easy to  spread infectious particles. The flight attendants are constantly in contact with the passengers. It is very important for them to perform an effective nasal cleansing after landed.

## New Students and New Soldiers

New college students and new soldiers come from everywhere in the nation. Different strains of cold viruses are brought to the new group of people. Most people catch the cold/flu when they breathe in tiny droplets from the coughs or sneezes of someone who has the cold/flu virus. It is also spread when you touch something with the virus on it and then touch your nose or eyes. It is truly your responsibility to perform an effective nasal cleansing to prevent cold virus infection during the risky time.

## How to Use NasalCare to Perform Nasal Cleansing

Here are the directions for using the NasalCare Kit:

A.   Basic Cleansing Procedures:

1) Wash your hands. Remove the clear dust cover, and then remove the cap from the bottle. Open one Nasal Rinse Mix packet and pour all the contents into the bottle.

2) Fill the bottle with lukewarm water (similar to your body temperature) to the 8-ounce (240 milliliter) line. Make sure the gasket is securely within the cap and the tube is tightly inserted into the small connector in the cap.

Screw the cap onto the bottle tightly. Shake the bottle several times to dissolve the mixture. To keep the solution from spilling out, use the tip of your finger to block the opening of the nostril fitting.

3) Bend forwards over a sink—like you would when brushing your teeth. Place the nostril fitting snugly into one nostril. Breathe through the mouth, not the nose, while performing nasal irrigation. Squeeze and release the bottle gently to allow the solution to flow into your nostril on one side, and let the washing solution flow out from the other nostril. Squeeze and release repeatedly about every half second. Doing so makes the cleansing process more efficient and relaxing. Do not squeeze the bottle all the way in one motion or squeeze it for too long. Otherwise, the hand pump will not function properly.

4)   Gently blow your nose to remove the mucus.

5)   Repeat steps 3 and 4 in the other nostril.

B.   Alternative Cleansing Procedures

During Step 3, if you find out your left and right nostril are not connected, you can let the solution run into your nostril and then flow out from your mouth; you just need to inhale through your nose. Then spit into the sink.

Even though your left and right nostrils are connected through the nasopharynx, you may still want to let the liquid run from the nostril to your mouth. This way, both your nasopharynx and oropharynx get cleansed.

Initially, some patients may be nervous about having water enter their nasal cavity, perhaps recalling unpleasant memories of having water enter their nose while swimming. However, since the NasalCare® solution has been carefully designed to suit the sensitive lining of the nose, nasal irrigation with NasalCare® is comfortable, even pleasant, as some patients have reported!

## The Most Complete Nasal Cleansing Procedure

To have a complete nasal cavity, nasopharynx and oropharynx cleansing, you are encouraged to try the following procedure after mastering the basic procedure.

1)  Gently pump the solution into one nostril, let about ¼ of the solution in the bottle to flow out from the other nostril; then gently blow your nose. This is to cleanse the left nasal passage, sinuses, the nasopharynx, and finally the right side of the nasal passage.

2)  Gently pump the solution into the other nostril, let the 2-ounce solution flow out from the opposite nostril, and then gently blow your nose. This is to cleanse the right nasal passage, sinuses, the nasopharynx from the other direction, and finally the left side of the nasal passage.

3) Gently pump the solution into the left side of the nostril. When you feel that side of the nasal cavity is full, inhale the liquid through your nose so the solution comes into your mouth. Spit it out into the sink. These two ounces are to cleanse the left nasal passage, left sinuses, nasopharynx, and then the left side of the oropharynx and the throat.

4)  Gently pump the solution into the right nostril; when you feel that side of the nasal cavity is full, inhale the liquid through your nose so the solution comes into your mouth. Spit it out into the sink. These two ounces are to cleanse the right nasal passage, right sinuses,

nasopharynx, and then the right side of the oropharynx and the throat.

## Removing Residual Water

It is common to have a small amount of liquid left in the nasal cavity, mainly in the maxillary sinuses, since the floor of this pair of sinuses is lower than the floor of the nasal cavity.

To drain the residual liquid from your sinuses, you can bend over, pointing your nose toward your knees, and then gently shake your head left to right a few times. Raise your head slowly. You will see some of the residual liquid has dropped out. You may repeat this action several more times to remove all the residual liquid.

## Maintenance After Each Use

After each nasal cleansing, fill the bottle with tap water and replace the gap. Pump water through it a few times so that the entire liquid passage is completely rinsed. Rinse the outside of the irrigator, especially the part that fits into the nostril, since that is the only piece to have touched your nose. Let all the rinsed parts air dry for the next use.

You may initially think that nasal irrigation doesn't seem very easy, as it takes a few steps before you actually use it. However, after just one use, you will see it is actually very simple and easy to do. Many users have shared that using the NasalCare® Nasal Irrigation Kit is easier than using neti pots.

## Anti-Inflammatory Drugs after Nasal Irrigation

After performing an effective nasal cleansing, the cold viruses are removed from your nasal cavity, and you can take any anti-inflammatory drug if your symptoms still bother you. There is no harm in suppressing inflammation now since the cold viruses are largely cleansed out. Suppressing inflammation with a drug will make you feel better more quickly. There is no interaction between nasal irrigation and any of the anti-inflammation drugs.

## You Can Use Other Methods to Further Help Reduce Symptoms and Speed Recovery

If you think chicken soup or vitamin C might have helped you to speed up the recovery process the last time you had a cold, you are encouraged to drink chicken soup or take vitamin C. You need the fluid and more vitamin C anyway during the infection period.

You can take zinc lozenges too, but not at the toxic level, which is more than 75 milligrams per day. With effective nasal irrigation, the need for zinc supplements is reduced. You don't need take such a high dose of zinc that could cause toxicity.

With regard to herbal supplements, that's your choice. If you know the herbal supplement is safe, you should feel free to take any of them.

## Physician's Help Is Needed for Any Viral Infection

For any viral infection, you need to seek professional medical help. The therapy discussed here is to cure colds is for adults and children at least five years of age, for practical reasons. In younger children, the Eustachian tubes are basically horizontal, so the ear and nasopharynx are at the same level. It could be easy for the liquid to run into the ear when performing nasal irrigation, which could increase the risk of an ear infection.

For infants and younger children who cannot perform nasal irrigation, the following complications can occur and a visit to a doctor will be necessary.

## Ear Infections

During the cold, children may experience a feeling of plugged ears and mild ear pain. This happens when mucus blocks the middle ear space behind the eardrum, just as the sinuses get congested with mucus. When bacteria grow in this mucus, this can cause an ear infection. If your child complains of ear pain or a plugged feeling, you should bring him or her to see a physician. Infants and very young children cannot tell you about ear pain, but they will be particularly fussy and feed and sleep poorly when dealing with an ear infection.

## Sinus Infections

A cold virus infection causes mucus accumulation, providing an ideal environment for bacterial growth. Signs of a sinus infection include Green nasal discharge for ten days or more and pain or pressure behind and around the eyes, forehead, and upper cheeks.

If you suspect that you or a family member has a sinus infection, please consult your doctor.

## Bronchitis

A productive cough is usually just part of the cold virus. However, if you also experience fever for more than five days, chest pains, and rapid breathing or wheezing, this could indicate bronchitis.

If these symptoms appear, you should seek your physician's advice.

## Pneumonia

This occurs when bacteria overgrow in the mucus down in the lungs. That is why it is important to cough up this mucus. Following are the signs that your child's cold and cough may have developed into pneumonia:

1)   Fever (over 101 degrees) more than five days, not just 99 or 100 degrees. However, if your child has other symptoms along with the fever, consult your doctor. Most, but not all, children with bacterial pneumonia will spike temperatures over 102º.

2)   Shortness of breath—Signs of this include rapid breathing, labored breathing, moving the shoulders up and down to assist in breathing, or sucking in below the ribs or at the base of the neck.

3)   Chest pains—your child will complain of a specific area of pain in the chest. In this case, it is best to seek your physician's advice.

# 11. Special Patients and Nasal Irrigation

Rhinoviruses cause over half of respiratory tract infections. Complications of rhinovirus infections, which include exacerbations of asthma, otitis media, sinusitis, and other pulmonary diseases, can be clinically important in certain populations.

It can be very challenging when cold viruses cause an infection during pregnancy. Using NasalCare to cleanse cold viruses out is a safe and effective therapy. This is not only a good practice for the mother, also protective for the fetus.

Below are several conditions which are strongly related to cold virus infection. Performing an effective nasal cleansing may help to reduce the severity or frequency of these diseases.

## Asthma Exacerbation by Cold Virus Infection

Numerous studies have demonstrated that upper respiratory tract infections with cold viruses trigger asthma attacks (flare ups).

Almost thirty years ago, the association between viral infections and the exacerbation of asthma in children was demonstrated, using tissue cultures and serological methods of detecting viruses. Subsequently, other studies using similar methods reported comparable findings in both adults and children. However, respiratory viruses, are difficult to detect by standard methods, and therefore, earlier studies may have underestimated the impact of viral infections on asthma-related wheezing.

Upon the development of highly sensitive laboratory methods, such as RT-PCR assays, they have been applied in studies investigating the relationship between viral infections and asthma severity. In a 1993 prospective study of 138 adults with asthma, Dr. Nicholson and his associates collected nose and throat swabs and blood samples and tried to coincide collections with either symptoms of acute upper respiratory tract infection or a worsening of asthma. Their study showed that 75 percent of cold viruses were associated with asthma attacks.

Dr. Johnston and colleagues performed a similar study in nine- to eleven-year-old children in 1995. Viruses were detected in 80 percent of reported episodes of asthma, with the rhinovirus identified most often. They also reported that the seasonal patterns of upper respiratory tract infection correlated with hospital admissions for asthma, but the relationship was stronger for pediatric than for adult admissions.

A study by Dr. Zhu and associates in 2009 went further in answering why rhinovirus infection triggers asthma attacks. It is well known in the medical community that nasal mucociliary clearance is a critical innate defense system responsible for clearing up invading pathogens, including bacteria and viruses. At the right amounts, mucus is beneficial, but too much mucus blocks the airways and can exacerbate disease symptoms. In their study, Dr. Zhu and colleagues found that both major and minor groups of rhinovirus induced mucus production in primary human epithelial cells and cell lines. This suggests that viral-induced mucus overproduction may contribute to virus-induced airway disease exacerbation, including asthma.

Since an asthma attack is a very serious condition, the authors encourage these patients to continue their asthma treatment under a physician's care. Since nasal cleansing is proven to remove cold viruses from the nasal cavity effectively, and can reduce the severity of nasal inflammation, patients with asthma are encouraged to perform nasal irrigation regularly, especially during the cold season. You may recall your asthma worsening when you had a cold. Now, you can perform nasal cleansing at the first signs of a cold. We predict that an effective nasal cleansing may help to reduce the frequency of flare-ups of asthma. A friend of ours has suffered from asthma for many years. After she used NasalCare® to perform nasal irrigation, her asthma flare-ups were reduced from seven times a week to one time a week. You can try to see if this result could be reproduced in your case.

There is no harm in the asthma patient performing nasal cleansing with NasalCare®. For the general population, the timely cure of a cold is important, but for asthma patients, the timely cure of a cold may be even more important. However, even if the frequency of your asthma attacks is significantly reduced, you should carry your inhaler all the time, or follow your doctor's suggestion.

## Sinusitis and Cold Virus Infection

Most cases of acute community-acquired bacterial sinusitis are believed to be secondary to a preceding viral upper-respiratory-tract infection. This view has been supported by many studies in which respiratory viruses were isolated from sinus aspirates of patients with acute community-acquired sinusitis. Sinus abnormalities were detected by magnetic resonance imaging (MRI) in volunteers with experimental rhinovirus colds and by computed tomography (CT) in patients with natural rhinovirus colds.

To understand the mechanism underlying viral sinusitis, a major question is whether sinus abnormalities are due to direct viral invasion or inflammatory events in adjacent areas in the nose. Dr. Frederick Hayden and associates conducted a study in 1997 to investigate if rhinovirus infection is closely related to sinus abnormality. Their study clearly supports the concept that viruses make people more vulnerable to bacterial infection of the maxillary sinuses. In natural colds, sinus abnormalities are observed by CT in over 85 percent of patients.

Since sinusitis is very common and patients with acute and chronic sinusitis have a poor quality of life, it is in their best interest to use NasalCare® to treat a cold whenever it occurs. Nasal irrigation has been recommended by the top ENTs in the country as the first line of therapy for treating chronic sinusitis; there will be even more benefit for these patients when they use the best nasal irrigation product available to treat their diseases.

## COPD and Cold Virus Infection

Respiratory viruses have been implicated as triggers that worsen chronic obstructive pulmonary disease (COPD). Human rhinovirus is the most common player in increasing the severity of symptoms, lung function changes, and inflammation in exacerbations of COPD. The changes in lower airway inflammation and lung function are more pronounced in proven rhinoviral and putative viral infections. Patients with severe COPD demonstrated greater rises in airway and systemic inflammation than those with milder forms of the disease. This suggests that the mixed nature of exacerbation severity is dependent not only on the nature of infective triggers but also on the inflammation status. Therefore, the patients with COPD need to pay more attention to viral infection.

Respiratory viral infection is an important trigger for the airway immune system. Rhinovirus can be isolated from lower airway samples and is associated with greater levels of inflammation than non-viral infections. Similarly, Dr. Jadwiga Wedzicha et al. have shown that colds are associated with more severe exacerbations of COPD. In their study, systemic inflammation, exacerbation symptoms of COPD, and lung function changes were all more severe when evidence for both bacterial and viral infection was present.

Furthermore, these exacerbations were associated with higher bacterial loads than when both pathogens were not present, which may suggest a synergistic interactive effect of viral infection, which allows greater proliferation of airway bacteria. Viral infection therefore may indirectly influence exacerbation severity by increasing the bacterial load in addition to the direct effects of the viral infection itself. While human rhinovirus is the most common virus identified at exacerbation and hence the target of investigation in their study, a number of other respiratory viruses have been identified in the airway during these events, for example coronavirus. The role of these other viral pathogens and atypical bacteria in exacerbation of COPD requires more investigation.

For patients with COPD, performing nasal irrigation with NasalCare® will provide great benefits. In addition, timely cleansing of cold viruses will stop these chain reactions caused by cold viruses, including the subsequent bacterial infection.

It is in the best interests of patients with COPD to use NasalCare to treat a cold as early as possible.

## Pregnancy and Cold Virus Infection

It is commonly known that the pregnant women are easy to catch a cold. Cold viruses have been linked to abnormalities in the fetus. Because of safety concerns for the fetus, pregnant women are particularly advised not to take some medicines. Nasal irrigation with NasalCare® can effectively remove cold viruses from the body without harming the fetus.

## Bacteria and Cold Viruses Mixed Infection

Cold virus infection damages the epithelium of the nasal cavity, which makes it easier to contract a bacterial infection. The mechanisms by which viral infection facilitate bacterial growth are likely to be complex. However, any disruption of the innate defenses of the respiratory epithelium in a lower airway colonized with bacteria may unsettle a fine balance between host immunity and bacterial numbers. Rhinoviral infection increases mucus production and neutrophilic inflammation. Furthermore, *in vitro* studies have shown that rhinoviral infection increases the susceptibility of epithelial cells to bacterial adherence, a key step in bacterial infection. Hence, through a number of mechanisms, viral infection may alter the immune environment and either allow proliferation of colonizing airway bacteria or a new pathogen to infect the lower airway.

## Bad Breath and Cold Virus Infection

Chronic bad breath is not just an oral hygiene issue; it is a disease needed to be treated by the joint efforts of ENT doctors and dentists, as bad breath is very closely related to post nasal drip, excess mucus, sinus problems, and your tonsils.

What is the main cause? Bacteria growth. Bacterial metabolism causes bad breath and sour, bitter, and metallic tastes. These bacteria are anaerobic (live without oxygen) and typically use the carbohydrates, fats and proteins in foods that we eat as fuel. However, under certain conditions, they will also start to break down the proteins found in mucus and phlegm.

Patients suffering from post nasal drip and sinus problems are more likely to have bad breath because when the bacteria use the mucus as a food source, they extract sulfur compounds from the proteins in mucus.

### Treatment of Bad Breath

For anyone suffering from excess mucus, sinus congestion and post nasal drip, there are several therapies:

(1)  Over-the-counter drugs

There are dozens of over-the-counter nasal decongestants and antihistamines, which can help relieve congestion. While these drugs dry up the sinuses and prevent mucus buildup, they also cause dry mouth, a likely side-effect of virtually all antihistamines. You should therefore be careful about using any antihistamine too frequently.

Even in cases where dry mouth is minimal, when you stop taking that medication the problem comes back, often worse than before. This is because in some cases, your body will actually develop a resistance to any antihistamines or nasal decongestants, especially nasal sprays because many sprays are habit forming.

(2)  Nasal irrigation as a natural healing

Performing an effective nasal irrigation can cleanse your sinuses, freeing them from excess mucus. For treating chronic sinusitis, top ENT physicians recognize that an effective nasal irrigation is the first line therapy. Nasal irrigation is the most effective method of eliminating post nasal drip and helping to control sinus infections. When you feel a sinus condition come on, or feel that you have persistent post-nasal drip and excess mucus, consistent daily use for ten days should result in an improved condition.

# Glossary

**Abdominal**: Relating to the abdomen, the belly, that part of the body that contains all of the structures between the chest and the pelvis. The abdomen is separated anatomically from the chest by the diaphragm, the powerful muscle spanning the body cavity below the lungs.

**Abdominal pain**: Pain in the belly (the abdomen). Abdominal pain can come from conditions affecting a variety of organs. The abdomen is an anatomical area that is bounded by the lower margin of the ribs above, the pelvic bone (pubic ramus) below, and the flanks on each side. Although abdominal pain can arise from the tissues of the abdominal wall that surround the abdominal cavity (the skin and abdominal wall muscles), the term abdominal pain generally is used to describe pain originating from organs within the abdominal cavity (from beneath the skin and muscles). These organs include the stomach, small intestine, colon, liver, gallbladder, and pancreas.

**Acetaminophen**: A pain reliever and fever reducer. Brand name: Tylenol. The exact mechanism of action of acetaminophen is not known. Acetaminophen relieves pain by elevating the pain threshold (that is, by requiring a greater amount of pain to develop before it is felt by a person). Acetaminophen reduces fever through its action on the heat-regulating center (the "thermostat") of the brain. Generic is available.

**Acquired**: Anything that is not present at birth but develops some time later. In medicine, the word "acquired" implies "new" or "added." An acquired condition is "new" in the sense that it is not genetic (inherited) and "added" in the sense that was not present at birth.

**Adenovirus**: A group of viruses responsible for a spectrum of respiratory disease as well as infection of the stomach/intestine (gastroenteritis), eyes (conjunctivitis), and bladder (cystitis) and rash. Adenovirus respiratory diseases include a form of the common cold, pneumonia, croup, and bronchitis. Patients with compromised immune systems are especially susceptible to severe complications of adenovirus infection. Acute respiratory disease (ARD), a disorder first recognized among military recruits during World War II, can be caused by adenovirus infections under conditions of crowding and stress.

**Aloe vera**: A short-stemmed plant with thick leaves with a soothing, viscous juice; leaves develop spiny margins with maturity; native to Mediterranean region; grown widely in tropics and as houseplants.

**Antihistamines**: Drugs that combat the histamine released during an allergic reaction by blocking the action of the histamine on the tissue. Since antihistamines do not stop the formation of histamine or the conflict between the antibody and antigen, they only protect tissues from some of the allergic reaction's effects. Antihistamines often cause mouth dryness and sleepiness. The "non sedating" antihistamines may be less effective.

**Asthma**: A chronic respiratory disease, often arising from allergies, that is characterized by sudden recurring attacks of labored breathing, chest constriction, and coughing.

**Bacteria**: Single-celled microorganisms which can exist either as independent (free-living) organisms or as parasites (dependent upon another organism for life).

**Buffer**: A buffer is a solution containing either a weak acid and its salt or a weak base and its salt, which is resistant to changes in pH.

**Chest pain**: There are many causes of chest pain. One is angina which results from inadequate oxygen supply to the heart muscle. Angina can be caused by coronary artery disease or spasm of the coronary arteries. Chest pain can also be due to a heart attack (coronary occlusion) and other important diseases such as, for example, dissection of the aorta and a pulmonary embolism. Do not try to ignore chest pain and "work (or play) though it." Chest pain is a warning to seek medical attention.

**Chills**: Feelings of coldness accompanied by shivering. Chills may develop after exposure to a cold environment or may accompany a fever.

**Chronic obstructive pulmonary disease (COPD)**: Any disorder that persistently obstructs bronchial airflow. COPD mainly involves two related diseases, chronic bronchitis and emphysema, which lead to the obstruction of airflow through the respiratory system. The condition is generally permanent and worsens over time.

**Citric acid**: A colorless translucent crystalline acid, principally derived by fermentation of carbohydrates or from lemon, lime, and pineapple juices.

**Conchae**: Any turbinate bone, especially in the nose.

**Common cold**: A viral upper respiratory tract infection. This contagious illness can be caused by many different types of viruses, and it is impossible for the body to build up resistance to all of them. This makes colds a frequent and recurring problem.

**Congestion**: An abnormal or excessive accumulation of a bodily fluid. Examples include nasal congestion (excess mucus and secretions in the air passages of the nose) seen with a common cold and congestion of blood in the lower extremities seen with some types of heart failure.

**Coronavirus**: One of a group of viruses, which look like a corona (halo) when viewed under a electron microscope. This appearance is due to an array of surface projections.

**Discharge**: The flow of fluid from a part of the body, such as the nose.

**Eustachian tube**: The tube that runs from the middle ear to the nasopharynx. Eustachian tube protects, aerates and drains the middle ear. Blockage of the Eustachian tube leads to inflammation of the middle ear. The Eustachian tube is also called the otopharyngeal tube (because it connects the ear to the pharynx) and the auditory tube (and in Latin, the tuba acustica, tuba auditiva, and tuba auditoria).

**Fatigue**: A condition characterized by a reduced work capacity and efficiency of accomplishment, usually accompanied by tiredness. Fatigue can come on suddenly or be chronic and persist.

**Flu**: Short for influenza. The flu is caused by viruses that infect the respiratory tract. Most people who get the flu recover completely in 1 to 2 weeks, but some people develop serious and potentially life-threatening medical complications, such as pneumonia. Much of the illness and death caused by influenza can be prevented by annual influenza vaccination.

**Hoarseness**: Hoarseness is a term referring to abnormal voice changes. Hoarseness may be manifested as a voice that sounds breathy, strained, rough, raspy, or a voice that has higher or lower pitch. There are many causes of hoarseness, including viral laryngitis, vocal cord nodules, laryngeal papillomas, gastroesophageal reflux-related laryngitis, and environmental irritants (such as tobacco smoking). An accumulation of fluid in the vocal cords associated with hoarseness has been termed Reinke's edema. Reinke's edema may occur as a result of cigarette smoking or voice abuse (prolonged or extended talking or shouting). Rarely, hoarseness results from serious conditions such as cancers of the head and neck region.

**Ibuprofen**: A non-steroidal anti-inflammatory drug (NSAID) commonly used to treat pain, swelling, and fever. Common brand names for Ibuprofen include Advil, Motrin, and Nuprin.

**Incubation period**: In medicine, the time from initial exposure to an infectious agent till the appearance of the first signs and symptoms of the disease.

**Isotonic**: When a solution has the same osmotic pressure (concentration) as serum, which has a normal value of  osmolality between 270–300 mOsm/kg water. Hypertonic: osmolality is higher than  300  mOsm/kg water; Hypotonic: osmolality is lower than 270 mOsm/kg water. See also "osmolality."

**Mucus**: A thick slippery fluid produced by the membranes lining certain organs such as the nose, mouth, throat, and vagina. Mucus is the Latin word for "a semifluid, slimy discharge from the nose." Note that *mucus* is a noun while the adjective is *mucous*.

**Nasal cavity**: The vaulted chamber that lies between the floor of the cranium and the roof of the mouth of higher vertebrates extending from the external nares to the pharynx, being enclosed by bone or cartilage and usually incompletely divided into lateral halves by the septum of the nose, and having its walls lined with mucous membrane that is rich in venous plexuses and ciliated in the lower part which forms the beginning of the respiratory passage and warms and filters the inhaled air and that is modified as sensory epithelium in the upper olfactory part.

**Nasal mucus**: A slippery, sometimes thick, fluid produced by the membranes lining the nose. Excessive nasal mucus underlies a runny nose.

**Onset**: In medicine, the first appearance of the signs or symptoms of an illness. See also "incubation period."

**Osmolality**: The concentration of a solution in terms of osmoles of solutes per kilogram of solvent. Serum osmolality is a measure of the number of dissolved particles per unit of water in serum. The fewer the particles of solute in proportion to the number of units of water (solvent), the less concentrated the solution. Measurement of the serum osmolality indicates the hydration status within the cells because the osmotic equilibrium is constantly maintained on both sides of the cell membrane. Water moves freely back and forth across the membrane in response to the osmolar pressure being exerted by the molecules of solute in the intracellular and extracellular fluids. The normal value for serum osmolality is 270–300 mOsm/kg water. See also "isotonic."

**Over-the-counter (OTC)**: A drug or a medical device that can be purchased by the consumer without a physician's prescription.

**Parainfluenza**: A disease due to an acute respiratory infection caused by a parainfluenza virus, usually occurring in children. It may present as anything from a relatively mild influenza-like illness to bronchitis, croup, and pneumonia.

**Pathogenesis**: The development of a disease. The origin of a disease and the chain of events leading to that disease.

**Pulmonary**: Having to do with the lungs.

**Resistance**: Opposition or the ability to withstand something. For example, some forms of staphylococcus are resistant to treatment with antibiotics.

**Respiratory syncytial virus (RSV)**: A virus that causes mild respiratory infections, colds, and coughs in adults, but can produce severe respiratory problems, including bronchitis and pneumonia in young children. Patients with compromised immune, cardiac or pulmonary systems are at high risk.

**Runny nose**: Rhinorrhea is the medical term for this common problem. From the Greek words "rhinos" meaning "of the nose" and "rhoia" meaning "a flowing."

**Saline**: Relating to salt. As an adjective, "saline" means "containing salt." As a noun, "saline" is a salt solution, often adjusted to the normal salinity of the human body.

**Sea salt**: It is produced by the evaporation of sea water and that contains sodium chloride and trace elements such as sulfur, magnesium, zinc, potassium, calcium, and iron.

**Secretion**: A process in which a gland or tissue produces a biochemical and releases it for use by the organism or for excretion.

**Sinus**: An air-filled cavity in a dense portion of a skull bone. There are four pairs of sinuses: the frontal sinuses, behind the forehead; the maxillary sinuses, behind the cheeks; the sphenoid sinuses, behind the maxillary sinuses; and the ethmoid sinuses, behind the eyes. They are lined by mucous-secreting cells.

**Sinusitis**: Inflammation of the membrane lining the sinuses, which are directly connected to the nasal cavities.

**Strep**: Very commonly used shortened form of Streptococcus, a very common and important group of bacteria.

**Strep throat**: Strep throat is an infection caused by a type of bacteria called streptococcus, which can lead to serious complications if not adequately treated.

**Syndrome**: A set of signs and symptoms that tend to occur together and which reflect the presence of a particular disease or an increased chance of developing a particular disease.

**TCID$_{50}$**: The 50 percent viral tissue culture infectious dose; the level of viruses needed to cause an infection in half of the inoculated cells.

**Vaccine:** A preparation of a weakened or killed pathogen (bacterium or virus), or of a portion of the pathogen's structure that, when administered through injection or inhalation, stimulates antibody production or cellular immunity against the pathogen. Since the pathogen used is either weakened or killed, or just a portion of the full structure, it is incapable of causing severe infection, though it may cause side effects.

**Virus**: An infectious agent smaller than a bacterium, which cannot grow or reproduce apart from a living cell. A virus invades living cells and uses their chemical machinery to stay alive and to replicate itself.

# Index

# References

Abadie WM, McMains KC, and Weitzel EK. Irrigation penetration of nasal delivery systems: A cadaver study. Int Forum Allergy Rhinol, 2011; 1:46-49.

Adam P, Stiffman M, and Blake RL. A Clinical Trial of Hypertonic Saline Nasal Spray in Subjects With the Cold or Rhinosinusitis. Arch Fam Med. 1998;7:39-43.

Alho OP, Karttunen R, and Karttunen TJ. Nasal mucosa in natural colds: effects of allergic rhinitis and susceptibility to recurrent sinusitis. Clin Exp Immu. 2004; 37 (2):366-72.

Ao HF, Wang Q, Jiang BF and He CY. Efficacy and Mechanism of Nasal Irrigation with a Hand Pump against Influenza and Non-Influenza Viral Upper Respiratory Tract Infection. Journal of Infectious Diseases and Immunity. 2011; Vol. 3(6):96-105.

Bachmann G, Hommel G, and Michel O: Effect of irrigation of the nose with isotonic salt solution on adult patients with chronic paranasal sinus disease. Eur Arch Otorhinolaryngol. 2000; 257(10): 537-41.

Baker DH. Iodine Toxicity and Its Amelioration. Exp Biol Med. 2004; 229:473–478.

Barrett BP, Brown RL, Locken K, et al. Treatment of the common cold with unrefined echinacea: a randomized, double-blind, placebo-controlled trial. Annals of Internal Medicine. 2002;137(12):939–946.

Benninger MS. Nasal Mucociliary Transport after Exposure to Swimming Pool Water. American Journal of Rhinology, 1994; 8(5): 207-209.

Boston M, Dobratz EJ, Buescher ES, and Darrow DH. Effects of Nasal Saline Spray on Human Neutrophils. Arch Otolaryngol Head Neck Surg. 2003;129:660-664.

Brown CL, Graham SM. Nasal irrigations: good or bad? Curr Opin Otolaryngol Head Neck Surg, 2004; 12(1):9-13.

Butler CC, Robling M, Prout H, et al. Management of suspected acute viral upper respiratory tract infection in children with intranasal sodium cromoglicate: a randomised controlled trial. The Lancet 2002; 359 (9324): 2153-2158.

Casale TB, Romero FA, and Spierings EL. Intranasal noninhaled carbon dioxide for the symptomatic treatment of seasonal allergic rhinitis. J Allergy Clin Immunol. 2008; 121(1):105-109.

Cate TR, Couch RB, and Johnson KM. Studies with rhinovirus in volunteers: production of illness, effect of naturally acquired antibody, and demonstration of a protective effect not associated with serum antibody. J Clin Invest 1964; 43:56-67.

Cazacu AC, Greer J, Taherivand M and Demmler GJ. Comparison of Lateral-Flow Immunoassay and Enzyme Immunoassay with Viral Culture for Rapid Detection of Influenza Virus in Nasal Wash Specimens from Children. J Clin Microbiology. 2003; 41(5): 2132-2134.

Chang EHE, Wong K, Philpott K, and Javer A. Sinus Irrigation Bottles: A Potential Source of Infection? Rhinology World Program, April 15-19, 2009, Page 47, ABSTRACT NUMBER 1653.

Chen Y, Hamati E, Lee PK et al. Rhinovirus Induces Airway Epithelial Gene Expression through Double-Stranded RNA and IFN-Dependent Pathways. Am J Respir Cell Mol Biol. 2006; 34(2): 192–203.

Chilvers MA, McKean M, and Rutman A. et al. The effects of coronavirus on human nasal ciliated respiratory epithelium. Eur Respir J 2001; 18:965-970.

Couch RB. Rhinoviruses. In: Fields Virology, third edition, edited by B.N. Fields, D.M. Knipe, P.M. Howley, et al. Lippincott –Raven Publishers, Philadelphia 1996; Chapter 23, pp.713-734.

Couch RB. The common cold: Control.  J Infect Dis 1984,150: 167-73.

Douglas RG Jr, Cate TR, Gerone JP, Couch RB. Quantitative rhinovirus shedding patterns in volunteers. Am Rev Respir Dis. 1966; 94:159-167.

Eby GA. Zinc lozenges as cure for the common cold – A review and hypothesis. Medical Hypotheses 2010; 74: 482–492.

Eby GA, Davis DR, and Halcomb WW. Reduction in duration of common colds by zinc gluconate lozenges in a double-blind study. Antimicrobial Agents Chemotherapy 1984;25:20-4.

Eccles R. Understanding the symptoms of the common cold and influenza. Lancet Infect Dis 2005;5: 718–725.

Falsey AR, Formica MA, Treanor JJ and Walsh EE. Comparison of Quantitative Reverse Transcription-PCR to Viral Culture for Assessment of Respiratory Syncytial Virus Shedding. J Clin Microbiology. 2003; 41(9): 4160–4165.

Feily A, Namazi MR. Aloe vera in dermatology: a brief review. G Ital Dermatol Venereol. 2009; 144(1):85-91.

Fendrick AM, Monto AS, Nitghtengale B and Sanes M. The Economic Burdon of Non-Influenza-Related Viral Respiratory Tract Infection in the United States. Arch Intern Med. 2003: 163:487-494.

Georgitis JW. Nasal hyperthermia and simple irrigation for perennial rhinitis. Changes in inflammatory mediators. Chest, 1994; 106:1487–92.

Gern GE, Mosser AG, and Swenson CA. Inhibition of Rhinovirus Replication In Vitro and In Vivo by Acid-Buffered Saline. The Journal of Infectious Diseases 2007; 195:1137–1143.

Gern JE, Dick EC, Lee WW, and Murray S. Rhinovirus enters but does not replicate inside monocytes and airway macrophages. J. Immunology, 1996; 156(2): 621-627.

Gern JE, Vrtis R, Grindle KA, Swenson C, and Busse WW. Relationship of upper and lower airway cytokines to outcome of experimental rhinovirus infection. Am J Respir Crit Care Med 2000;162:2226–2231.

Godfrey JC, Sloane B, Smith DS, et al. Zinc gluconate and the common cold: A controlled clinical study. J Int Med Res 1992;20:234-46.

Griego SD, Weston CB, Adams JL. et al. Role of p38 Mitogen-Activated Protein Kinase in Rhinovirus-Induced Cytokine Production by Bronchial Epithelial Cells. The Journal of Immunology. 2000; 165: 5211–5220.

Gwaltney JM Jr. The common cold. In: Mandell GL, Bennett JE, Dolin R, eds. Mandell, Douglas and Bennett's

Principles and Practice of Infectious Diseases. 4[th]ed. New York: Churchill Livingstone, 1995:561-566.

Gwaltney JM, Hendley JO, Simon G, and Jordon WS. Rhinovirus infections in an industrial population. I. The occurrence of illness.. N Engl J Med 1966;275:1261-1268.

Gwaltney JM and Ruckert RR. Rhinovirus. In: Richmann DD, Whitley RJ, Hayden FG, eds. Clinical Virology. NY: Churchill Livingstone, 1997:1025-1047.

Hall CB and Douglas RJ. Clinically useful method for the isolation of respiratory syncytial virus, Journal of Infectious Diseases, 1975; 131: 1-5.

Hall CB and ouglas, R.J. Quantitative shedding patterns of respiratory syncytial virus in infants, Journal of Infectious Diseases, 1975; 132: 151-156.

Hall CB, Geiman JM, Breese BB, and Douglas RJ: Parainfluenza virus infections in children: Correlation of shedding with clinical manifestations, *Journal of Pediatrics*, 1977; 91: 194-198.

Harkema J, Carey S, and Wagner JG. The Nose Revisited: A Brief Review of the Comparative Structure, Function, and Toxicological Pathology of the Nasal Epithelium. Toxicological Pathology, 2006; 34:252–269.

Hauptman G and Ryan MW. The effect of saline solutions on nasal patency and mucociliary clearance in rhinosinusitis patients. Otolaryngol Head Neck Surg. 2007; 137(5):815-21.

Heatley DG, McConnell KE, Kille TL, Leverson GE. Nasal irrigation for the alleviation of sinonasal symptoms, Otolaryngol Head Neck Surg. 2001;125(1):44-48.

Hemila H. Vitamin C and the common cold. British Journal of Nutrition. 1992; 61, 3-16.

Holgate ST, Davies DE, Puddicombe S. et al. Mechanisms of airway epithelial damage: epithelial-mesenchymal interactions in the pathogenesis of asthma. Eur Respir J 2003; 22(Suppl. 44): 24s–29s.

Jackson GG and Muldoon RL. Viruses causing common respiratory infection in man. I. Rhinoviruses. J Infect Dis 1973; 127:328-355.

Jackson JL, Lesho E, and Peterson C. Zinc and the common cold: A meta-analysis revisited. J Nutr 2000; 130(5S Suppl):1512S-1015S.

Jakiela B, Brockman-Schneider R and Amineva S et al. Basal Cells of Differentiated Bronchial Epithelium Are More Susceptible to Rhinovirus Infection. Am J Respir Cell Mol Biol 2008; 38: 517–523.

Johnston SL. Overview of Virus-induced Airway Disease. The Proceedings of the American Thoracic Society 2005; 2:150-156.

Johnston SL, Papi A, Bates PJ et al. Low Grade Rhinovirus Infection Induces a Prolonged Release of IL-8 in Pulmonary Epithelium. The Journal of Immunology. 1998; 160: 6172–6181.

Kaliner M. Treatment of Sinusitis in the Next Millennium. Allergy & Asthma Proceedings. 1998;19:181.

Kaul P, Biagioli MC and Singh I. Rhinovirus-Induced Oxidative Stress and Interleukin-8 Elaboration Involves p47-phox but Is Independent of Attachment to Intercellular Adhesion Molecule–1 and Viral Replication. The Journal of Infectious Diseases 2000;181:1885–1890.

Kaul P, Singh I and Turner RB. Effect of Nitric Oxide on Rhinovirus Replication and Virus-Induced Interleukin-8 Elaboration. AM J RESPIR CRIT CARE MED 1999;159:1193–1198.

Korant BD and Butterworth BE. Inhibition by zinc of rhinovirus protein cleavage: Interaction of zinc with capsid polypeptides. J Virol 1976; 18:298-306.

Korant BD, Kauer JC, and Butterworth BE. Zinc ions inhibit replication of rhinoviruses. Nature 1974; 248:588-590.

Lavigne F, Tulic MK, Gagnon J, and Hamid Q. Selective irrigation of the sinuses in the management of chronic rhinosinusitis refractory to medical therapy: a promising start. J Otolaryngol-Head Neck Surg. 2004; 33(1):10-16.

Lee N, Chan PKS, Hui DSC et al. Viral Loads and Duration of Viral Shedding in Adult Patients Hospitalized with Influenza. The Journal of Infectious Diseases 2009; 200:492–500.

Liu J. Nasal-nasopharyngeal cleaning system. US Patent 6238377, Issued on May 29, 2001.

Liu J. Nasal-nasopharyngeal cleaning system. US Patent 6736792, Issued on May 18, 2004.

Liu J. and Zhang L. The unique solutions for nasal irrigation.  China Patent granted on February 14, 2007, Patent Number ZL2004 10024220.4.

Liu J. and Zhang L. A unique device to deliver the cleanse liquid to nasal and sinus cavities. China Patent granted on October 11, 2006, Patent Number ZL200520086805.9.

Manning SC: Pediatric Sinusitis. Otolaryngologic Clinics of North America. 1993; 26,4:623-637.

Meltzer EO, Hamilos DL, Hadley JA et al. Rhinosinusitis: Developing guidance for clinical trials. J. Allergy and Clinical Immunology 2006; 118(5): S17-S61.

Message SD and Johnston SL. Host defense function of the airway epithelium in health and disease: clinical background. J of Leukocyte Biology. 2004; 75(1): 5-17.

Michel O. Nasal irrigation in case of rhinosinusitis. Laryngorhinootologie. 2006; 85(6):448-58.

Mossad SB, Macknin ML, Medendorp SV, and Mason P. Zinc gluconate lozenges for treating the common cold. A randomized, double-blind, placebo-controlled study. Ann Intern Med 1996; 125:81-88.

Murray CS, Simpson A, and Custovic A. Allergens, Viruses, and Asthma Exacerbations. Proc Am Thorac Soc 2004; vol 1. pp 99–104.

Nsouli TM, et al.  Long-term use of nasal saline irrigation: Harmful or helpful? ACAAI, 2009; Abstract O32.

Olson DE, Rasgon BM, and Hilsinger RL. Radiographic comparison of three methods for nasal saline irrigation. Laryngoscope 2002; 112:1394–1398.

Panagiotopoulos G, Naxakis S, Papavasilious A, et al. Decreasing Nasal Mucus Ca+++ Improves Hyposmia. Rhinology. 2005; 43(2):130-134.

Papsin B and McTavish A. Saline nasal irrigation. Can Family Physician. 2003; 49:168-173.

Pitkaranta A, Arruda E, Malmberg H, and Hayden FG. Detection of Rhinovirus in Sinus Brushings of Patients with Acute Community-Acquired Sinusitis by Reverse Transcription-PCR. J. Clin Microbiology 1997; 35: 1791–93.

Pynnonen MA, Mukerji SS, Kim HM, Adams ME, and Terrell JE. Nasal Saline for Chronic Sinonasal Symptoms, A Randomized Controlled Trial. Arch Otolaryngol Head Neck Surg. 2007; 133(11):1115-1120.

Rabago D et al. Efficacy of daily saline nasal irrigation among patients with sinusitis: a randomized controlled trial. J Family Practice. 2003; 51(12): 1049-55.

Rabago D, Barrett B, Marchand L, Maberry R, and Mundt M. Qualitative Aspects of Nasal Irrigation Use by Patients With Chronic Sinus Disease in a Multimethod Study Annals of Family Medicine 2006; 4:295-301.

Rabago D, et al. The efficacy of hypertonic saline nasal irrigation for chronic sinonasal symptoms. Otolaryngol Head Neck Surg. 2005; 133(1):3-8.

Rabago D, Guerard E, Bukstein D. Nasal irrigation for chronic sinus symptoms in patients with allergic rhinitis, asthma, and nasal polyposis.WMJ. 2008; 107(2):69-75.

Rabone SJ and Saraswati SB: Acceptance and effects of nasal lavage in volunteer woodworkers. Occup Med (Lond), 1999; 49:365-369.

Rachelevsky GS, Slavin RG, and Wald ER. Sinusitis: Acute, Chronic and Manageable. Patient Care. 1997; 131:4.

Ravizza R and Fornadley J. Irrigation of the Nose Helps Prevent Colds. The 50th Scientific Assembly of the American

Academy of Family Physicians. San Francisco, Sept 21, 1998.

Rider TH, Zook CE, Boettcher TL, Wick ST, and Pancoast JS et al. Broad-Spectrum Antiviral Therapeutics. PLoS ONE 2011; 6(7): e22572. doi:10.1371/.

Scheid DC and Hamm RM. Acute bacterial rhinosinusitis in adults: part II. Treatment. Am Fam Physician. 2004; 70(9):1642, 1645.

Scott C. Pediatric sinusitis, Manning. In: Inflammatory Diseases of the Sinuses. Otolaryngologic Clinics of North America. 1993; 26:623-638.

Scott EJ and Heath GF. Factors Affecting the Growth of Rhinovirus 2 in Suspension Cultures of L 132 Cells. J. Gen. Virology 1970; 6:5-24.

Shah SA, Sander CS and White CM. Evaluation of echinacea for the prevention and treatment of the common cold: a meta-analysis. The Lancet Infectious Diseases. 2007; 7(7): 473-480.

Shaman J. Why more flu during winter season? http://blogs.discovermagazine.com/80beats/2009/02/10/scientists-solve-the-mystery-of-flu-season/

Shoseyov D, et al. Treatment with hypertonic saline versus normal saline nasal wash of pediatric chronic sinusitis. J Allergy Clin Immunol. 1998; 101(5): 602-605.

Slapak I, Skoupá J, Strnad P, and Horník P. Efficacy of isotonic nasal wash (seawater) in the treatment and prevention of rhinitis in children. Arch Otolaryngol Head Neck Surg. 2008; 134(1):67-74.

Talbot AR, Herr MH, and Parsons DS. Mucociliary clearance and buffered hypertonic saline solution. Laryngoscope 1997; 107:500-503.

Tano L and Tano K. A Daily Nasal Spray with Saline Prevents Symptoms of Rhinitis. Acta Oto-laryngologica, 2004; 124(9):1059-1062.

Taylor JA, Weber W, and Standish L. Efficacy and Safety of Echinacea in Treating Upper Respiratory Tract Infections in Children. JAMA. 2003;290(21):2824-2830.

Tomooka, LT, Murphy C, and Davidson TM. Clinical Study and Literature Review of Nasal Irrigation. The Laryngoscope. 2000; 110(7):1189–1193.

Tsao CH, Chen LC, Yeh KW and Huang JL. Concomitant Chronic Sinusitis Treatment in Children With Mild Asthma. The Effect on Bronchial Hyper-responsiveness. CHEST 2003; 123:757–764.

Turetsky BT, Glass CA, Abbazia J. et al. Reduced Posterior Nasal Cavity Volume: A Gender-Specific Neurodevelopmental Abnormality in Schizophrenia. Schizophr Res. 2007; 93(1-3): 237–244.

Turner RB, Bauer R, Woelkart K, Hulsey TC et al. An Evaluation of Echinacea angustifolia in Experimental Rhinovirus Infections. N Engl J Med 2005; 353:341-348.

Wedzicha JA and Donaldson GC. Exacerbations of Chronic Obstructive Pulmonary Disease. RESPIRATORY CARE. 2003; 48(12):1204-1213.

Welch KC, Cohen MB, Doghramji LL. et al. Clinical correlation between irrigation bottle contamination and clinical outcomes in post-functional endoscopic sinus surgery patients. Am J Rhinol Allergy 2009; 23, 401–404.

Wilkinson TMA, Hurst JR, Perera WR et Al. Effect of Interactions between Lower Airway Bacterial and Rhinoviral Infection in Exacerbations of COPD. CHEST 2006; 129:317–324.

Wormald PJ, Cain T, Oates L, Hawke L, and Wong I. A comparative study of three methods of nasal irrigation. Laryngoscope, 2004; 114:2224-2227.

Yu H, Dong Z, and Yang Z. Molecular biological study of aloe vera in the treatment of experimental allergic rhinitis in rat. Lin Chuang Er Bi Yan Hou Ke Za Zhi. 2002; 16(5):229-31.

Zeiger RS and Schatz M. Chronic Rhinitis: A Practical Approach to Diagnosis and Treatment. Immunology & Allergy Practice. 1982; 4(4):26-35.

Zeiger RS. Prospects for ancillary treatment of rhinosinusitis in the 1990's. J Allergy Clin Immunol. 1992; 90:478.

Zhu L, Lee PK, Lee WM et al. Rhinovirus-Induced Major Airway Mucin Production Involves a Novel TLR3-EGFR–Dependent Pathway. Am J Respir Cell Mol Biol 2009; 40: 610–619.

# About the Authors

Dr. James Z. Liu is a trained physician specializing in prevention and epidemiology of infectious diseases in Shandong University School of Preventive Medicine in 1982, and a doctor of philosophy (PhD) in Human Nutrition at the Pennsylvania State University in 1993. He has been a medical research scientist for thirty years with both academic institutions and pharmaceutical companies. During his early academic career, Dr. Liu published thirty-two peer-reviewed medical research articles and received numerous medical research awards from the central government, national professional societies, and academia. While working for the pharmaceutical industry, Dr. Liu authored twelve US patents, created and developed a number of new healthcare products. He has led multiple functional teams to conduct clinical trials for a number of top pharmaceutical companies during the last seventeen years. Currently at TechWorld Medicals, Dr. Liu continues his innovations and transforms medical sciences into practical technologies, and plays instrumental roles for gaining products approval/registration in US FDA and China SFDA.

Dr. Lilly Zhang has over 25 years of experience in medical research and drug development rewarded by over 50 publications, patents, and distinguished awards. She received her Ph.D. in Cell, Molecular & Neuroscience from University of Hawaii, finished her postdoctoral training at National Institutes of Health (NIH) where she later was promoted to a senior staff fellow. At NIH, she cloned a number of genes involved in regulation of gene expression by retinoids, carotenoid, hormones and growth factors during carcinogenesis, epidermal cell proliferation, differentiation and aging. She has given presentations at national and international conferences as well highly prestigious institutions.

Before co-founding TechWorld Corporation in 1998, she was the Senior Project Leader at P&G where she managed several important research projects, including programs for hair growth, weight loss, and fatigue relief. Her contributions were recognized by numerous distinguished awards and patents. Later, she lead the team at TWC to find a better solution for allergic rhinitis after suffering from the disease herself and then seeing her daughter suffer. She convinced from her personal experience and research that nasal allergies, sinusitis, colds and flu can be effectively prevented and treated by simply removal of harmful offenders inhaled from the air. Dr. Zhang has led the company with vision, innovation, understanding, and transforms advanced technologies and insights into new products. Under her strong leadership, the Research and Development Department has developed over 10 medical and healthcare products approved/registered by US FDA and/or China SFDA.

Dr. Liu's and Dr. Zhang's main interest is in developing novel devices, methods and practical approaches to prevent and treat common diseases. Collaborating with other skilled individuals, Dr. Liu and Dr. Zhang led the team to have designed, manufactured, and tested the OTC medical devices for treatment of a variety of disorders.

One of these medical devices is the NasalCare® Nasal Irrigation System. This system was the only winner of the "Best New Product Award" at the "2010 ECRM Cough & Cold and Allergy Conference" voted by professions across North America. A recent international clinical study demonstrates that using NasalCare® Nasal Irrigation System three times a day can dramatically reduce the severity and shorten the duration of the common cold and influenza (Ao et al 2011).

The clinical study verified what Dr. Liu originally hypothesized when he filed the U.S. patent application in 1997: physically removing viruses from nasal and nasopharyngeal cavities can be an effective method to treat and prevent infectious diseases, like the common cold. This new book will help to revolutionize how we treat the common cold.

Dr. Liu declared a war against common cold on October 28, 2011. We hopes all members of the global village will be actively participating in the fight to win the war.